History of the Great Plague

Compiled by

Kiera Mccune

Scribbles

Year of Publication 2018

ISBN : 9789352979295

Book Published by

Scribbles

(An Imprint of Alpha Editions)

email - alphaedis@gmail.com

Produced by: PediaPress GmbH
Limburg an der Lahn
Germany
http://pediapress.com/

Contents

Black Death Migration

Black Death migration

The Black Death was one of the most devastating pandemics in human history, resulting in the deaths of an estimated 75 to 200 million people in Eurasia and peaking in Europe from 1346 to 1353. Its migration followed the sea and land trading routes of the medieval world. This migration has been studied for centuries as an example of how the spread of contagious diseases is impacted by human society and economics.

The disease is caused by *Yersinia pestis*, which is enzootic (commonly present) in populations of ground rodents in Central Asia. Morelli et al. (2010) reported the origin of the plague bacillus to be in China. An older theory places the first cases in the steppes of Central Asia, and others, such as the historian Michael W. Dols, argue that the historical evidence concerning epidemics in the Mediterranean and specifically the Plague of Justinian point to a probability that the Black Death originated in Central Asia,[1] where it then became entrenched among the rodent population.[2]

Nevertheless, from Central Asia it was carried east and west along the Silk Road, by Mongol armies and traders making use of the opportunities of free passage within the Mongol Empire offered by the Pax Mongolica. It was reportedly first introduced to Europe at the trading city of Caffa in the Crimea in 1347. After a protracted siege, during which the Mongol army under Jani Beg was suffering the disease, they catapulted the infected corpses over the city walls to infect the inhabitants.[3] The Genoese traders fled, bringing the plague by ship into Sicily and the south of Europe, whence it spread.

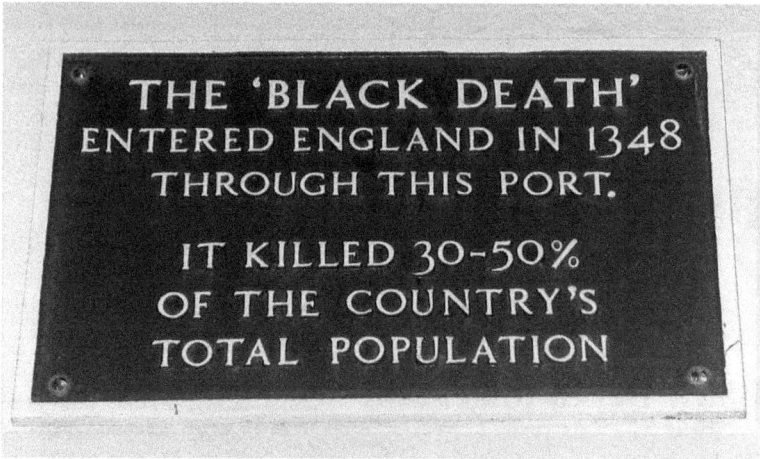

Figure 1: *Plaque in Weymouth, England*

Preexisting conditions

Regardless of its origin, it is clear that several preexisting conditions such as war, famine, and weather contributed to the severity of the Black Death. In China, the 13th century Mongol conquest disrupted farming and trading, and led to widespread famine. The population dropped from approximately 120 to 60 million.[4] The 14th century plague is estimated to have killed 1/3 of the population of China.Wikipedia:Citation needed

In Europe, the Medieval Warm Period ended sometime towards the end of the 13th century, bringing harsher winters and reduced harvests. In the years 1315 to 1317 a catastrophic famine, known as the Great Famine, struck much of North-West Europe. The famine came about as the result of a large population growth in the previous centuries, with the result that, in the early 14th century the population began to exceed the number that could be sustained by productive capacity of the land and farmers.

In Northern Europe, new technological innovations such as the heavy plough and the three-field system were not as effective in clearing new fields for harvest as they were in the Mediterranean because the north had poor, clay-like soil. Food shortages and skyrocketing prices were a fact of life for as much as a century before the plague. Wheat, oats, hay, and consequently livestock, were all in short supply, and their scarcity resulted in hunger and malnutrition. The result was a mounting human vulnerability to disease, due to weakened immune systems.

The European economy entered a vicious circle in which hunger and chronic, low-level debilitating disease reduced the productivity of labourers, and so the grain output was reduced, causing grain prices to increase. This situation was worsened when landowners and monarchs like Edward III of England (r. 1327–1377) and Philip VI of France (r. 1328–1350), out of a fear that their comparatively high standard of living would decline, raised the fines and rents of their tenants.[5] Standards of living then fell drastically, diets grew more limited, and Europeans as a whole experienced more health problems.

Heavy rains in autumn 1314 began several years of cold and wet winters. The already weak harvests of the north suffered and the seven-year famine ensued. The Great Famine was the worst in European history, reducing the population by at least ten percent. Records recreated from dendrochronological studies show a hiatus in building construction during the period, as well as a deterioration in climate.

This was the economic and social situation in which the predictor of the coming disaster, a typhoid (Infected Water) epidemic, emerged. Many thousands died in populated urban centres, most significantly Ypres. In 1318 a pestilence of unknown origin, sometimes identified as anthrax, targeted the animals of Europe, notably sheep and cattle, further reducing the food supply and income of the peasantry.

Asian outbreak

The scenario that would place the first outbreak in central Asia agrees with the first reports of outbreaks in China in the early 1330s. The plague struck the Chinese province of Hubei in 1334. On the heels of the European epidemic, a more widespread disaster occurred in China during 1353–1354. Chinese accounts of this wave of the disease record a spread to eight distinct areas: Hubei, Jiangxi, Shanxi, Hunan, Guangdong, Guangxi, Henan, and Suiyuan,[6] throughout the Mongol and Chinese empires. Historian William McNeill noted that voluminous Chinese records on disease and social disruption survive from this period, but no one has studied these sources in depth.[7]

It is probable that the Mongols and merchant caravans inadvertently brought the plague from central Asia to the Middle East and Europe. The plague was reported in the trading cities of Constantinople and Trebizond in 1344.

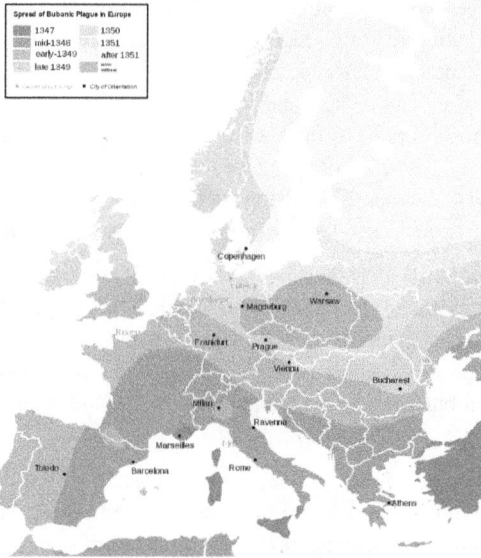

Figure 2: *The Black Death rapidly spread along
the major European sea and land trade routes*

European outbreak

In October 1347, a fleet of Genoese trading ships fleeing Caffa reached the
port of Messina in Sicily.[8] By the time the fleet reached Messina, all the crew
members were either infected or dead. It is presumed that the ships also carried
infected rats and/or fleas. Some ships were found grounded on shorelines, with
no one aboard remaining alive.

Looting of these lost ships also helped spread the disease. From there, the
plague spread to Genoa and Venice by the turn of 1347–1348.

From Italy the disease spread northwest across Europe, striking France, the
Crown of Aragon, the Crown of Castile, Portugal and England by June 1348,
then turned and spread east through Germany and Scandinavia from 1348 to
1350. It was introduced in Norway in 1349 when a ship landed at Askøy,
then proceeded to spread to Bjørgvin (modern Bergen). Finally it spread to
north-western Russia in 1351; however, the plague largely spared some parts
of Europe, including the Kingdom of Poland, isolated parts of Belgium and the
Netherlands, Milan and the modern-day France-Spain border.

At Siena, Agnolo di Tura wrote:

'They died by the hundreds, both day and night, and all were thrown in ...
ditches and covered with earth. And as soon as those ditches were filled,
more were dug. And I, Agnolo di Tura ... buried my five children with my
own hands ... And so many died that all believed it was the end of the
world. "

Middle Eastern outbreak

The plague struck various countries in the Middle East during the pandemic,
leading to serious depopulation and permanent change in both economic and
social structures. As it spread to western Europe, the disease also entered the
region from southern Russia. By autumn 1347, the plague reached Alexandria
in Egypt, probably through the port's trade with Constantinople, and ports
on the Black Sea. During 1348, the disease travelled eastward to Gaza, and
north along the eastern coast to cities in Lebanon, Syria, and Palestine, including Ashkelon, Acre, Jerusalem, Sidon, Damascus, Homs, and Aleppo. In
1348–49, the disease reached Antioch. The city's residents fled to the north,
most of them dying during the journey, but the infection had been spread to
the people of Asia Minor.

Mecca became infected in 1349. During the same year, records show the
city of Mawsil (Mosul) suffered a massive epidemic, and the city of Baghdad
experienced a second round of the disease. In 1351, Yemen experienced an
outbreak of the plague. This coincided with the return of King Mujahid of
Yemen from imprisonment in Cairo. His party may have brought the disease
with them from Egypt.

Recurrence

In England, in the absence of census figures, historians propose a range of pre-
incident population figures from as high as 7 million to as low as 4 million in
1300, and a post-incident population figure as low as 2 million.[9] By the end
of 1350 the Black Death had subsided, but it never really died out in England
over the next few hundred years: there were further outbreaks in 1361–62,
1369, 1379–83, 1389–93, and throughout the first half of the 15th century.
The plague often killed 10% of a community in less than a year—in the worst
epidemics, such as at Norwich in 1579 and Newcastle in 1636, as many as 30 or
40%. The most general outbreaks in Tudor and Stuart England, all coinciding
with years of plague in Germany and the Low Countries, seem to have begun
in 1498, 1535, 1543, 1563, 1589, 1603, 1625, and 1636.

The plague repeatedly returned to haunt Europe and the Mediterranean
throughout the 14th to 18th centuries, and still occurs in isolated cases today.

The plague of 1575–77 claimed some 50,000 victims in Venice. In 1634, an outbreak of plague killed 15,000 Munich residents. Late outbreaks in central Europe include the Italian Plague of 1629–1631, which is associated with troop movements during the Thirty Years' War, and the Great Plague of Vienna in 1679. About 200,000 people in Moscow died of the disease from 1654 to 1656. Oslo was last ravaged in 1654. In 1656 the plague killed about half of Naples' 300,000 inhabitants. Amsterdam was ravaged in 1663–1664, with a mortality given as 50,000.

The Great Plague of London in 1665–1666 is generally recognized as one of the last major outbreaks.

A plague epidemic that followed the Great Northern War (1700–1721, Sweden v. Russia and allies) wiped out almost 1/3 of the population in the region.Wikipedia:Citation needed An estimated one-third of East Prussia's population died in the plague of 1709–1711. The plague of 1710 killed two-thirds of the inhabitants of Helsinki. An outbreak of plague between 1710 and 1711 claimed a third of Stockholm's population.

During the Great Plague of 1738, the epidemic struck again, this time in Eastern Europe, spreading from Ukraine to the Adriatic Sea, then onwards by ship to infect some in Tunisia. The destruction in several cities in what is now Romania (such as Timişoara) was formidable, claiming tens of thousands of lives.

Theories

Theories of the Black Death

Theories of the Black Death are a variety of explanations that have been advanced to explain the nature and transmission of the Black Death (1347–69). A number of epidemiologists and since the 1980s have challenged the traditional view that the Black Death was caused by plague based on the type and spread of the disease. The confirmation in 2010 and 2011 that *Yersinia pestis* DNA was associated with a large number of plague sites has renewed focus on plague as the leading hypothesis, but has not yet led to a final resolution of all these questions.

Bubonic plague theory

Several possible causes have been advanced for the Black Death; the most prevalent is the bubonic plague theory. Efficient transmission of *Yersinia pestis* is generally thought to occur only through the bites of fleas whose mid guts become obstructed by replicating *Y. pestis* several days after feeding on an infected host. This blockage results in starvation and aggressive feeding behaviour by fleas that repeatedly attempt to clear their blockage by regurgitation, resulting in thousands of plague bacteria being flushed into the feeding site, infecting the host. However, modelling of epizootic plague observed in prairie dogs, suggests that occasional reservoirs of infection such as an infectious carcass, rather than "blocked fleas" are a better explanation for the observed epizootic behaviour of the disease in nature.

One hypothesis about the epidemiology—the appearance, spread, and especially disappearance—of plague from Europe is that the flea-bearing rodent reservoir of disease was eventually succeeded by another species. The black rat (*Rattus rattus*) was originally introduced from Asia to Europe by trade, but was subsequently displaced and succeeded throughout Europe by the bigger brown rat (*Rattus norvegicus*). The brown rat was not as prone to transmit the

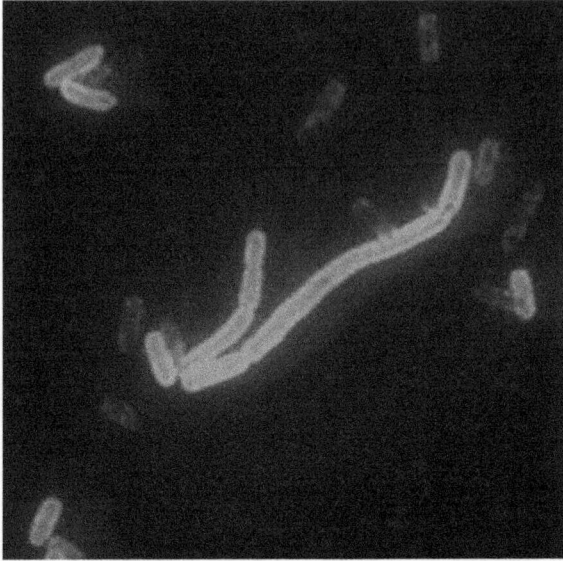

Figure 3: *Yersinia pestis seen at 2000× magnification. This bacterium, carried and spread by fleas, is generally thought to have been the cause of millions of deaths.*

germ-bearing fleas to humans in large die-offs due to a different rat ecology. The dynamic complexities of rat ecology, herd immunity in that reservoir, interaction with human ecology, secondary transmission routes between humans with or without fleas, human herd immunity, and changes in each might explain the eruption, dissemination, and re-eruptions of plague that continued for centuries until its unexplained disappearance.

Signs and symptoms of the three plagues

The three forms of plague brought an array of signs and symptoms to those infected. The septicaemic plague is a form of "blood poisoning", and pneumonic plague is an airborne plague that attacks the lungs before the rest of the body. The classic sign of bubonic plague was the appearance of buboes in the groin, the neck, and armpits, which oozed pus and bled. Most victims died within four to seven days after infection. When the plague reached Europe, it first struck port cities and then followed the trade routes, both by sea and land.

The bubonic plague was the most commonly seen form during the Black Death, with a mortality rate of thirty to seventy-five percent and symptoms including fever of 38–41 °C (101–105 °F), headaches, painful aching joints, nausea and vomiting, and a general feeling of malaise. Of those who contracted the bubonic plague, four out of five died within eight days.[10] Pneumonic plague was the second most commonly seen form during the Black Death, with a mortality rate of ninety to ninety-five percent. Symptoms included fever, cough, and blood-tinged sputum. As the disease progressed, sputum became free flowing and bright red and death occurred within 2 days. Septicemic plague was the least common of the three forms, with a mortality rate close to one hundred percent. Symptoms were high fevers and purple skin patches (purpura due to DIC). Both pneumonic and septicemic plague can be caused by flea bites when the lymph nodes are overwhelmed. In this case they are referred to as *secondary* forms of the disease.

David Herlihy[11] identifies from the records another potential sign of the plague: freckle-like spots and rashes. Sources from Viterbo, Italy refer to "the signs which are vulgarly called *lenticulae*", a word which bears resemblance to the Italian word for freckles, *lentiggini*. These are not the swellings of buboes, but rather "darkish points or pustules which covered large areas of the body".

Molecular evidence for *Y. pestis*

In 2000, Didier Raoult and others reported finding *Y. pestis* DNA by performing a "suicide PCR" on tooth pulp tissue from a fourteenth-century plague cemetery in Montpellier. Drancourt and Raoult reported similar findings in a 2007 study.

However, other researchers argued the study was flawed and cited contrary evidence. In 2003, Susan Scott of the University of Liverpool argued that there was no conclusive reason to believe the Montpellier teeth were from Black Death victims. Also in 2003, a team led by Alan Cooper from Oxford University tested 121 teeth from sixty-six skeletons found in 14th century mass graves, including well-documented Black Death plague pits in East Smithfield and Spitalfields. Their results showed no genetic evidence for *Y. pestis*, and Cooper concluded that though "[w]e cannot rule out *Yersinia* as the cause of the Black Death ...right now there is no molecular evidence for it.". Other researchers argued that those burial sites where *Y. pestis* could not be found had nothing to do with the Black Death in the first place

In October 2010 the journal *PLoS Pathogens* published a paper Haensch et al. (2010) by a multinational team that investigated the role of *Yersinia pestis* in the Black Death. The paper detailed the results of new surveys that combined ancient DNA analyses and protein-specific detection which were used to find DNA and protein signatures specific for *Y. pestis* in human skeletons from widely distributed mass graves in northern, central and southern Europe that were associated archaeologically with the Black Death and subsequent resurgences. The authors concluded that this research, together with prior analyses from the south of France and Germany

"...ends the debate about the etiology of the Black Death, and unambiguously demonstrates that *Y. pestis* was the causative agent of the epidemic plague that devastated Europe during the Middle Ages."

Significantly, the study also identified two previously unknown but related clades (genetic branches) of the *Y. pestis* genome that were associated with distinct medieval mass graves. These were found to be ancestral to modern isolates of the modern *Y. pestis* strains Orientalis and Medievalis, suggesting that these variant strains (which are now presumed to be extinct) may have entered Europe in two distinct waves.

The presence of *Y. pestis* during the Black Death and its phylogenetic placement was definitely established in 2011 with the publication of a *Y. pestis* genome using new amplification techniques used on DNA extracts from teeth from over 100 samples from the East Smithfield burial site in London.

Surveys of plague pit remains in France and England indicate that the first variant entered Europe through the port of Marseilles around November 1347 and spread through France over the next two years, eventually reaching England in the spring of 1349, where it spread through the country in three successive epidemics. However, surveys of plague pit remains from the Netherlands town of Bergen op Zoom showed that the *Y. pestis* genotype responsible for the pandemic that spread through the Low Countries from 1350 differed from that found in Britain and France, implying that Bergen op Zoom (and possibly other parts of the southern Netherlands) was not directly infected from England or France in AD 1349, suggesting that a second wave of plague infection, distinct from those in Britain and France, may have been carried to the Low Countries from Norway, the Hanseatic cities, or another site.

Alternative explanations

Evidence against *Y. pestis*

Although *Y. pestis* as the causitive agent of plague is widely accepted, recent scientific and historical investigations have led some researchers to doubt the long-held belief that the Black Death was an epidemic of bubonic plague.

While *Y. pestis* was in some samples collected from grave sites in various burial sites across Europe, many skeletons did not yield the DNA. The fact that bubonic plague DNA was present does not necessarily mean that bubonic plague was the cause of death; the individual could possibly have survived a bout of bubonic plague and died of another disease agent. *Y. pestis* might well have been the cause of death, but since archaeologists have often specifically sought evidence of *Y. pestis*, other important information is potentially neglected. While rats were present in major sea ports across Europe, the evidence for rats in rural communities in Northern Europe is scanty. The fact that the epidemiology of the Black Death and its rapid spread does not match modern bubonic plague is an indication that all possibilities should be considered, even in the case that the epidemic was caused by bubonic plague[12]

In 1984, Graham Twigg published *The Black Death: A Biological Reappraisal*, where he argued that the climate and ecology of Europe and particularly England made it nearly impossible for rats and fleas to have transmitted bubonic plague. Combining information on the biology of *Rattus rattus*, *Rattus norvegicus*, and the common fleas *Xenopsylla cheopis* and *Pulex irritans* with modern studies of plague epidemiology, particularly in India, where the *R. rattus* is a native species and conditions are nearly ideal for plague to be spread, Twigg concludes that it would have been nearly impossible for *Yersinia pestis* to have been the causative agent of the plague, let alone its explosive spread across Europe. Twigg also shows that the common theory of entirely pneumonic spread does not hold up. He proposes, based on a reexamination of the evidence and symptoms, that the Black Death may actually have been an epidemic of pulmonary anthrax caused by *Bacillus anthracis*.

In 2002, Samuel K. Cohn published the controversial article, "The Black Death: End of the Paradigm". In the article Cohn argues that the medieval and modern plagues were two distinct diseases differing in their symptoms, signs, and epidemiologies. Cohn asserts that the agent causing the bubonic plague, *Yersinia pestis*, "was first cultured at Hong Kong in 1894." In turn, the medieval plague that struck Europe, according to Cohn, was not the bubonic plague carried by fleas on rats as traditionally viewed by scientists and historians alike.

Cohn's argument that medieval plague was not rat-based is supported by his claims that the modern and medieval plagues hit in different seasons (a claim supported in a 2009 article by Mark Welford and Brian Bossak), had unparalleled cycles of recurrence, and varied in the manner in which immunity was acquired. The modern plague reaches its peak in seasons with high humidity and a temperature of between 50 °F (10 °C) and 78 °F (26 °C), as rats' fleas thrive in this climate. In comparison, the Black Death is recorded as hitting in periods where rats' fleas could not survive, i.e. hot Mediterranean summers above 78 °F (26 °C). In terms of recurrence, the Black Death on average did not resurface in an area for between five and fifteen years after it hit. Contrastingly, modern plagues often hit an affected area yearly for an average of eight to forty years. Last, Cohn presents evidence displaying that individuals gained immunity to the Black Death during the fourteenth century, unlike the modern plague. He states that in 1348 two-thirds of those suffering from plague died in comparison to one-twentieth by 1382. Statistics contrastingly display that immunity to the modern plague has not been acquired.

In the Encyclopedia of Population, he points to five major weaknesses in this theory:

- very different transmission speeds — the Black Death was reported to have spread 385 km in 91 days (4.23 km/day) in 664, compared to 12–15 km a year for the modern bubonic plague, with the assistance of trains and cars
- difficulties with the attempt to explain the rapid spread of the Black Death by arguing that it was spread by the rare pneumonic form of the disease — in fact this form killed less than 0.3% of the infected population in its worst outbreak (Manchuria in 1911)
- different seasonality — the modern plague can only be sustained at temperatures between 10 and 26 °C and requires high humidity, while the Black Death occurred even in Norway in the middle of the winter and in the Mediterranean in the middle of hot dry summers
- very different death rates — in several places (including Florence in 1348) over 75% of the population appears to have died; in contrast the highest mortality for the modern bubonic plague was 3% in Bombay in 1903
- the cycles and trends of infection were very different between the diseases — humans did not develop resistance to the modern disease, but resistance to the Black Death rose sharply, so that eventually it became mainly a childhood disease

Cohn also points out that while the identification of the disease as having buboes relies on accounts of Boccaccio and others, they described buboes, abscesses, rashes and carbuncles occurring all over the body, the neck or behind the ears. In contrast, the modern disease rarely has more than one bubo, most commonly in the groin, and is not characterised by abscesses, rashes and carbuncles. This difference, he argues, ties in with the fact that fleas caused the modern plague and not the Black Death. Since flea bites do not usually reach beyond a person's ankles, in the modern period the groin was the nearest lymph node that could be infected. As the neck and the armpit were often infected during the medieval plague, it appears less likely that these infections were caused by fleas on rats.[13]

Ebola-like virus

In 2001, Susan Scott and Christopher Duncan, respectively a demographer and zoologist from Liverpool University, proposed the theory that the Black Death might have been caused by an Ebola-like virus, not a bacterium. Their rationale was that this plague spread much faster and the incubation period was much longer than other confirmed *Y. pestis*–caused plagues. A longer period of incubation will allow carriers of the infection to travel farther and infect more people than a shorter one. When the primary vector is humans, as opposed to birds, this is of great importance. Epidemiological studies suggest the disease was transferred between humans (which happens rarely with *Yersinia pestis* and very rarely for *Bacillus anthracis*), and some genes that determine immunity to Ebola-like viruses are much more widespread in Europe than in other parts of the world. Their research and findings are thoroughly documented in *Biology of Plagues*.[14] More recently the researchers have published computer modeling demonstrating how the Black Death has made around 10% of Europeans resistant to HIV.

Anthrax

In a similar vein, historian Norman Cantor, in *In the Wake of the Plague: The Black Death and the World It Made* (2001), suggests the Black Death might have been a combination of pandemics including a form of anthrax, a cattle murrain. He cites many forms of evidence including: reported disease symptoms not in keeping with the known effects of either bubonic or pneumonic plague, the discovery of anthrax spores in a plague pit in Scotland, and the fact that meat from infected cattle was known to have been sold in many rural English areas prior to the onset of the plague. The means of infection varied widely, with infection in the absence of living or recently dead humans in Sicily (which speaks against most viruses). Also, diseases with similar symptoms were generally not distinguished between in that period (see *murrain* above), at least not in the Christian world; Chinese and Muslim medical records can be expected to yield better information which however only pertains to the specific disease(s) which affected these areas.

Cutaneous anthrax infection in humans shows up as a boil-like skin lesion that eventually forms an ulcer with a black center (eschar), often beginning as an irritating and itchy skin lesion or blister that is dark and usually concentrated as a black dot. Cutaneous infections generally form within the site of spore penetration between two and five days after exposure. Without treatment about 20% of cutaneous skin infection cases progress to toxemia and death. Respiratory infection in humans initially presents with cold or flu-like symptoms for several days, followed by severe (and often fatal) respiratory collapse. Historical mortality was 92%.[15] Gastrointestinal infection in humans is most often caused by eating anthrax-infected meat and is characterized by serious gastrointestinal difficulty, vomiting of blood, severe diarrhea, acute inflammation of the intestinal tract, and loss of appetite. After the bacteria invades the bowel system, it spreads through the bloodstream throughout the body, making more toxins on the way.

Counter-arguments

Historians who believe that the Black Death was indeed caused by bubonic plague have put forth several counterarguments.

The uncharacteristically rapid spread of the plague could be due to respiratory droplet transmission, and low levels of immunity in the European population at that period. Historical examples of pandemics of other diseases in populations without previous exposure, such as smallpox and tuberculosis transmitted by aerosol amongst Native Americans, show that the first instance of an epidemic spreads faster and is far more virulent than later instances among the descendants of survivors, for whom natural selection has produced characteristics that are protective against the disease.

A 2012 report from the University of Bergen acknowledges that *Y. pestis* could have been the cause of the pandemic, but states that the epidemiology of the disease is different, most importantly the rapid spread and the lack of rats in Scandinavia and other parts of Northern Europe. *R. rattus* was present in Scandinavian cities and ports at the time of the Black Death but was not found in small, inland villages. Based on archaeological evidence from digs all over Norway, the black rat population was present in sea ports but remained static in the cold climate and would only have been sustained if ships continually brought black rats and that the rats would be unlikely to venture across open ground to remote villages. It argues that while healthy black rats are rarely seen, rats suffering from bubonic plague behave differently from healthy rats; where accounts from warmer climates mention rats falling from roofs and walls and piling high in the streets, Samuel Pepys, who described trifling observations and events of the London plague of 1665 in great detail, makes no mention of sick or dead rats, nor does Absalon Pederssøn in his diary, which contains detailed descriptions of a plague epidemic in Bergen in 1565. Ultimately, Hufthammer and Walløe offer the possibility of human fleas and lice in place of rats.[16]

University of Oslo researchers concluded that *Y. pestis* was likely carried over the Silk Road via fleas on giant gerbils from Central Asia during intermittent warm spells.[17,18]

Michael McCormick, a historian offering the idea that bubonic plague was indeed the source of the Black Death, explains how archaeological research has confirmed that the black or "ship" rat was indeed present in Roman and medieval Europe. Also, the DNA of *Y. pestis* has been identified in the teeth of the human victims, the same DNA which has been widely believed to have come from the infected rodents. He does not deny the point that there exists a pneumonic expression of *Y. pestis* transmitted by human-to-human contact, but he states that this does not spread as easily as previous historians have imagined.

The rat, according to him, is the only plausible agent of transmission that could have led to such a wide and quick spread of the plague. This is because of rats' proclivity to associate with humans and the ability of their blood to withstand very large concentrations of the bacillus. When rats died, their fleas (which were infected with bacterial blood) found new hosts in the form of humans and animals. The Black Death tapered off in the eighteenth century, and according to McCormick, a rat-based theory of transmission could explain why this occurred. The plague(s) had killed a large portion of the human host population of Europe and dwindling cities meant that more people were isolated, and so geography and demography did not allow rats to have as much contact with Europeans. Greatly curtailed communication and transportation systems due to the drastic decline in human population also hindered the replenishment of devastated rat colonies.Wikipedia:Please clarify

Consequences

Consequences of the Black Death

The **consequences of the Black Death** are the short-term and long-term effects of the Black Death on human populations across the world. They include a series of various biological, social, economic, political and religious upheavals which had profound impacts on the course of world history, especially European history. Often referred to as simply "The Plague", the Black Death was one of the most devastating pandemics in human history, peaking in Europe between 1347 and 1350 with an estimated one-third of the continent's population ultimately succumbing to the disease. Historians estimate that it reduced the total world population from 450 million to between 350 and 375 million. In most parts of Europe, it took nearly 80 years for population sizes to recover, and in some areas more than 150 years.

From the perspective of many of the survivors, however, the impact of the plague may have been ultimately favorable, as the massive reduction of the workforce meant their labor was suddenly in higher demand. R.H. Hilton has argued that those English peasants who survived found their situation to be much improved. For many Europeans, the 15th century was a golden age of prosperity and new opportunities. The land was plentiful, wages high, and serfdom had all but disappeared. A century later, as population growth resumed, the lower classes again faced deprivation and famine.[19,20]

Death toll

Figures for the death toll vary widely by area and from source to source, and estimates are frequently revised as historical research brings new discoveries to light. Most scholars estimate that the Black Death killed between 75 and 200 million people in the 14th century, at a time when the entire world population was still less than 500 million. Even where the historical record is considered reliable, only rough estimates of the total number of deaths from the plague are possible.

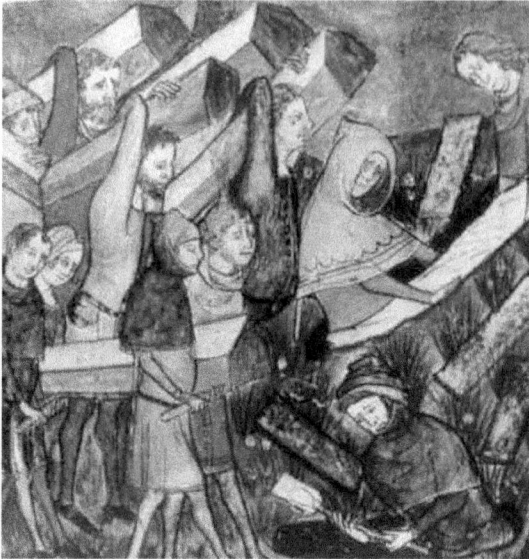

Figure 4: *Citizens of Tournai bury plague victims. Detail of a miniature from "The Chronicles of Gilles Li Muisis" (1272–1352). Bibliothèque royale de Belgique, MS 13076-77, f. 24v.*

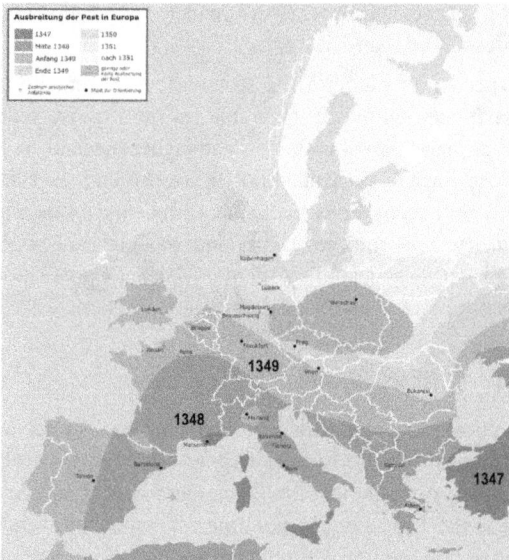

Figure 5: *The spread of the "Black Death" through Europe from 1347 to 1351*

Europe

Europe suffered an especially significant death toll from the plague. Modern estimates range between roughly one-third and one-half of the total European population in the five-year period of 1347 to 1351, during which the most severely affected areas may have lost up to 80 percent of the population.[21] Contemporary chronicler Jean Froissart, incidentally, estimated the toll to be one-third, which modern scholars consider less an accurate assessment than an allusion to the Book of Revelation meant to suggest the scope of the plague.[22] Deaths were not evenly distributed across Europe, with some areas affected very little while others were all but entirely depopulated.[23]

The Black Death hit the culture of towns and cities disproportionately hard, although rural areas (where most of the population lived at the time) were also significantly affected. Larger cities were the worst off, as population densities and close living quarters made disease transmission easier. Cities were also strikingly filthy, infested with lice, fleas, and rats, and subject to diseases caused by malnutrition and poor hygiene.[24] Florence's population was reduced from 110,000–120,000 inhabitants in 1338 to 50,000 in 1351. Between 60 and 70 percent of Hamburg's and Bremen's populations died. In Provence, Dauphiné, and Normandy, historians observe a decrease of 60 percent of fiscal hearths. In some regions, two-thirds of the population was annihilated. In the town of Givry, in the Bourgogne region of France, the local friar, who used to note 28 to 29 funerals a year, recorded 649 deaths in 1348, half of them in September. About half of Perpignan's population died over the course of several months (only two of the eight physicians survived the plague). Over 60 percent of Norway's population died between 1348 and 1350. London may have lost two-thirds of its population during the 1348–49 outbreak; England as a whole may have lost 70 percent of its population, which declined from 7 million before the plague to 2 million in 1400.[25]

A few rural areas, especially in Eastern Poland and Lithuania, had such low populations and were so isolated that the plague made little progress there. Other places, including parts of Hungary, the Brabant region, Hainaut, and Limbourg (in modern Belgium), as well as Santiago de Compostela, were unaffected for unknown reasons. Some historians[26] have assumed that the presence of resistant blood groups in the local population helped them resist infection, although these regions were touched by the second plague outbreak in 1360–63 (the "little mortality") and later during the numerous resurgences of the plague (in 1366–69, 1374–75, 1400, 1407, etc.). Other areas which escaped the plague were isolated in mountainous regions (e.g. the Pyrenees).

All social classes were affected, although the lower classes, living together in unhealthy places, were most vulnerable. Alfonso XI of Castile was the only

European monarch to die of the plague, but Peter IV of Aragon lost his wife, his daughter, and a niece in six months. Joan of England, daughter of Edward III, died in Bordeaux on her way to Castile to marry Alfonso's son, Pedro. The Byzantine Emperor lost his son, while in the Kingdom of France, Joan of Navarre, daughter of Louis X *le Hutin* and Margaret of Burgundy, was killed by the plague, as well as Bonne of Luxembourg, the wife of the future John II of France.

Asia

Estimates of the demographic impact of the plague in Asia are based on population figures during this time and estimates of the disease's toll on population centers. The most severe outbreak of plague in the Chinese province of Hubei in 1334 claimed up to 80 percent of the population.Wikipedia:Citation needed China had several epidemics and famines from 1200 to the 1350s and its population decreased from an estimated 125 million to 65 million in the late 14th century.

The precise demographic impact of the disease in the Middle East is very difficult to calculate. Mortality was particularly high in rural areas, including significant areas of Gaza and Syria. Many rural people fled, leaving their fields and crops, and entire rural provinces are recorded as being totally depopulated. Surviving records in some cities reveal a devastating number of deaths. The 1348 outbreak in Gaza left an estimated 10,000 people dead, while Aleppo recorded a death rate of 500 per day during the same year. In Damascus, at the disease's peak in September and October 1348, a thousand deaths were recorded every day, with overall mortality estimated at between 25 and 38 percent. Syria lost a total of 400,000 people by the time the epidemic subsided in March 1349. In contrast to some higher mortality estimates in Asia and Europe, scholars such as John Fields of Trinity College in Dublin believe the mortality rate in the Middle East was less than one-third of the total population, with higher rates in selected areas.

Social, environmental, and economic effects

Because 14th-century healers were at a loss to explain the cause of the Black Death, many Europeans ascribed supernatural forces, earthquakes and malicious conspiracies, among other things, as possible reasons for the plague's emergence. No one in the 14th century considered rat control a way to ward off the plague, and people began to believe only God's anger could produce such horrific displays of suffering and death. Giovanni Boccaccio, an Italian writer and poet of the era, questioned whether it was sent by God for their correction, or that it came through the influence of the heavenly bodies. Christians accused Jews of poisoning public water supplies in an effort to ruin European civilization. The spreading of this rumor led to complete destruction of entire Jewish towns, and was simply caused by suspicion on part of the Christians, who noticed that the Jews had lost fewer lives to the plague due to their hygienic practices. In February 1349, 2,000 Jews were murdered in Strasbourg. In August of the same year, the Jewish communities of Mainz and Cologne were exterminated.[27]

Where government authorities were concerned, most monarchs instituted measures that prohibited exports of foodstuffs, condemned black market speculators, set price controls on grain, and outlawed large-scale fishing. At best, they proved mostly unenforceable. At worst, they contributed to a continent-wide downward spiral. The hardest hit lands, like England, were unable to buy grain abroad from France because of the prohibition and from most of the rest of the grain producers because of crop failures from shortage of labour. Any grain that could be shipped was eventually taken by pirates or looters to be sold on the black market. Meanwhile, many of the largest countries, most notably England and Scotland, had been at war, using up much of their treasury and exacerbating inflation. In 1337, on the eve of the first wave of the Black Death, England and France went to war in what would become known as the Hundred Years' War. Malnutrition, poverty, disease and hunger, coupled with war, growing inflation and other economic concerns made Europe in the mid-14th century ripe for tragedy.

Europe had been overpopulated before the plague, and a reduction of 30 to 50 percent of the population could have resulted in higher wages and more available land and food for peasants because of less competition for resources.[28] Historian Walter Scheidel contends that waves of plague following the initial outbreak of the Black Death had a leveling effect that changed the ratio of land to labor, reducing the value of the former while boosting that of the latter, which lowered economic inequality by making landowners and employers less well off while improving the lot of the workers. He states that "the observed improvement in living standards of the laboring population was rooted in the suffering and premature death of tens of millions over the course of several generations." This leveling effect was reversed by a "demographic recovery that resulted in renewed population pressure." In 1357, a third of property in London was unused due to a severe outbreak in 1348–49. However, for reasons that are still debated, population levels declined after the Black Death's first outbreak until around 1420 and did not begin to rise again until 1470, so the initial Black Death event on its own does not entirely provide a satisfactory explanation to this extended period of decline in prosperity. See Medieval demography for a more complete treatment of this issue and current theories on why improvements in living standards took longer to evolve.

Impact on peasants

The great population loss brought favourable results to the surviving peasants in England and Western Europe. There was increased social mobility, as depopulation further eroded the peasants' already weakened obligations to remain on their traditional holdings. Seigneurialism never recovered. Land was plentiful, wages high, and serfdom had all but disappeared. It was possible to move about and rise higher in life. Younger sons and women especially benefited. As population growth resumed, however, the peasants again faced deprivation and famine.[29]

In Eastern Europe, by contrast, renewed stringency of laws tied the remaining peasant population more tightly to the land than ever before through serfdom. Sparsely populated Eastern Europe was less affected by the Black Death and so peasant revolts were less common in the fourteenth and fifteenth centuries, not occurring in the east until the sixteenth through nineteenth centuries.

Furthermore, the plague's great population reduction brought cheaper land prices, more food for the average peasant, and a relatively large increase in per capita income among the peasantry, if not immediately, in the coming century. Since the plague left vast areas of farmland untended, they were made available for pasture and put more meat on the market; the consumption of meat and dairy products went up, as did the export of beef and butter from the Low Countries, Scandinavia and northern Germany. However, the upper class often attempted to stop these changes, initially in Western Europe, and more forcefully and successfully in Eastern Europe, by instituting sumptuary laws. These regulated what people (particularly of the peasant class) could wear, so that nobles could ensure that peasants did not begin to dress and act as a higher class member with their increased wealth. Another tactic was to fix prices and wages so that peasants could not demand more with increasing value. In England, Statute of Labourers 1351 was enforced, meaning no peasant could ask for more wages than in 1346.[30] This was met with varying success depending on the amount of rebellion it inspired; such a law was one of the causes of the 1381 Peasants' Revolt in England.

The rapid development of the use was probably one of the consequences of the Black Death, during which many landowning nobility died, leaving their realty to their widows and minor orphans.Wikipedia:Citation needed

Impact on urban workers

In the wake of the drastic population decline brought on by the plague, wages shot up and laborers could move to new localities in response to wage offers. Local and royal authorities in Western Europe instituted wage controls. These governmental controls sought to freeze wages at the old levels before the Black

Death. Within England, for example, the Ordinance of Labourers, enacted in 1349, and the Statute of Labourers, enacted in 1351, restricted both wage increases and the relocation of workers. If workers attempted to leave their current post, employers were given the right to have them imprisoned. The Statute was poorly enforced in most areas, and farm wages in England on average doubled between 1350 and 1450,[31] although they were static thereafter until the end of the 19th century.

Cohn, comparing numerous countries, argues that these laws were not primarily designed to freeze wages. Instead, he says the energetic local and royal measures to control labor and artisans' prices was a response to elite fears of the greed and possible new powers of lesser classes that had gained new freedom. Cohn says the laws reflect the anxiety that followed the Black Death's new horrors of mass mortality and destruction, and from elite anxiety about manifestations such as the flagellant movement and the persecution of Jews, Catalans, and beggars.[32]

Labour-saving innovation

By 1200, virtually all of the Mediterranean basin and most of northern Germany had been deforested and cultivated. Indigenous flora and fauna were replaced by domestic grasses and animals and domestic woodlands were lost. With depopulation, this process was reversed. Much of the primeval vegetation returned, and abandoned fields and pastures were reforested.

The Black Death encouraged innovation of labour-saving technologies, leading to higher productivity. There was a shift from grain farming to animal husbandry. Grain farming was very labor-intensive, but animal husbandry needed only a shepherd and a few dogs and pastureland.

Plague brought an eventual end of Serfdom in Western Europe. The manorial system was already in trouble, but the Black Death assured its demise throughout much of western and central Europe by 1500. Severe depopulation and migration of the village to cities caused an acute shortage of agricultural laborers. Many villages were abandoned. In England, more than 1300 villages were deserted between 1350 and 1500. Wages of labourers were high, but the rise in nominal wages following the Black Death was swamped by post-Plague inflation, so that real wages fell.

Labor was in such a short supply that Lords were forced to give better terms of tenure. This resulted in much lower rents in western Europe. By 1500, a new form of tenure called copyhold became prevalent in Europe. In copyhold, both a Lord and peasant made their best business deal, whereby the peasant got use of the land and the Lord got a fixed annual payment and both possessed a copy of the tenure agreement. Serfdom did not end everywhere. It lingered in parts of Western Europe and was introduced to Eastern Europe after the Black Death.

There was change in the inheritance law. Before the plague, only sons and especially the elder son inherited the ancestral property. Post plague all sons as well as daughters started inheriting property.

Persecutions

Renewed religious fervor and fanaticism came in the wake of the Black Death. Some Europeans targeted "groups such as Jews, friars, foreigners, beggars, pilgrims",[33] lepers[34] and Romani, thinking that they were to blame for the crisis.

Differences in cultural and lifestyle practices also led to persecution. As the plague swept across Europe in the mid-14th century, annihilating more than half the population, Jews were taken as scapegoats, in part because better hygiene among Jewish communities and isolation in the ghettos meant that Jews were less affected.[35,36] Accusations spread that Jews had caused the disease by deliberately poisoning wells.[37,38] European mobs attacked Jewish settlements across Europe; by 1351, 60 major and 150 smaller Jewish communities had been destroyed, and more than 350 separate massacres had occurred.

According to Joseph P. Byrne, women also faced persecution during the Black Death. Muslim women in Cairo became scapegoats when the plague struck.[39] Byrne writes that in 1438, the sultan of Cairo was informed by his religious lawyers that the arrival of the plague was Allah's punishment for the sin of fornication and that in accordance with this theory, a law was set in place stating that women were not allowed to make public appearances as they may tempt men into sin. Byrne describes that this law was only lifted when "the wealthy complained that their female servants could not shop for food."

Religion

The Black Death hit the monasteries very hard because of their proximity with the sick who sought refuge there. This left a severe shortage of clergy after the epidemic cycle. Eventually the losses were replaced by hastily trained and inexperienced clergy members, many of whom knew little of the rigors of their predecessors. New colleges were opened at established universities, and the training process sped up.[40] The shortage of priests opened new opportunities for laywomen to assume more extensive and more important service roles in the local parish.[41]

Flagellants practiced self-flogging (whipping of oneself) to atone for sins. The movement became popular after the Black Death. It may be that the flagellants' later involvement in hedonism was an effort to accelerate or absorb God's

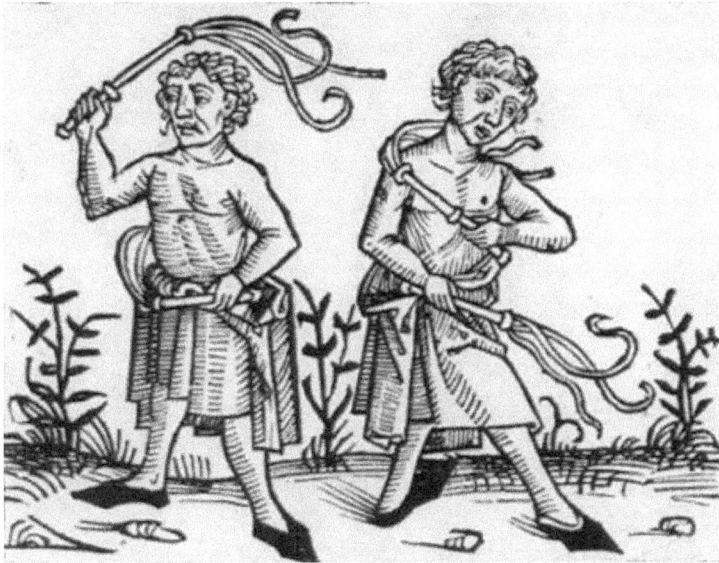

Figure 6: *Woodcut of flagellants (Nuremberg Chronicle, 1493)*

wrath, to shorten the time with which others suffered. More likely, the focus of attention and popularity of their cause contributed to a sense that the world itself was ending and that their individual actions were of no consequence.

Reformers rarely pointed to failures on the part of the Church in dealing with the catastrophe.[42]

Cultural impact

The Black Death had a profound impact on art and literature. After 1350, European culture in general turned very morbid. The general mood was one of pessimism, and contemporary art turned dark with representations of death. The widespread image of the "dance of death" showed death (a skeleton) choosing victims at random. Many of the most graphic depictions come from writers such as Boccaccio and Petrarch.[43] Peire Lunel de Montech, writing about 1348 in the lyric style long out of fashion, composed the following sorrowful *sirventes* "Meravilhar no·s devo pas las gens" during the height of the plague in Toulouse:

> They died by the hundreds, both day and night, and all were thrown in ... ditches and covered with earth. And as soon as those ditches were filled, more were dug. And I, Agnolo di Tura ... buried my five children with my

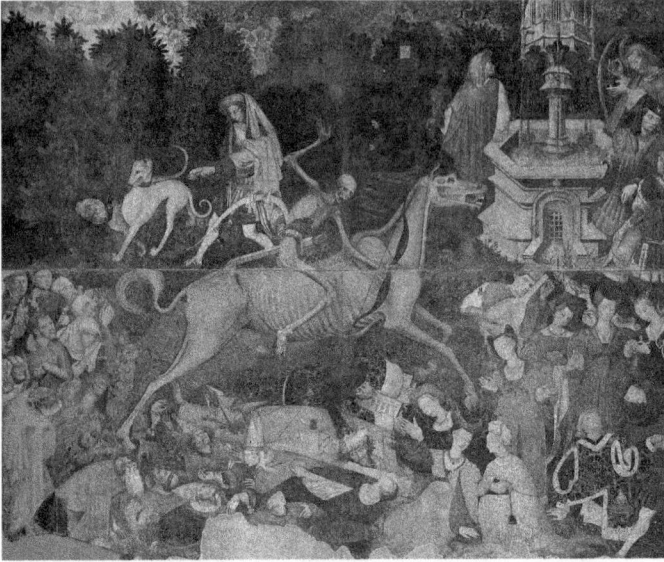

Figure 7: *The Triumph of Death (1446)*

own hands ... And so many died that all believed it was the end of the world.

Boccaccio wrote:

How many valiant men, how many fair ladies, breakfast with their kinfolk and the same night supped with their ancestors in the next world! The condition of the people was pitiable to behold. They sickened by the thousands daily, and died unattended and without help. Many died in the open street, others dying in their houses, made it known by the stench of their rotting bodies. Consecrated churchyards did not suffice for the burial of the vast multitude of bodies, which were heaped by the hundreds in vast trenches, like goods in a ships hold and covered with a little earth.[44]

Medicine

Although the Black Death highlighted the shortcomings of medical science in the medieval era, it also led to positive changes in the field of medicine. As described by David Herlihy in *The Black Death and the Transformation of the West,* more emphasis was placed on "anatomical investigations" following the Black Death.[45] How individuals studied the human body notably changed, becoming a process that dealt more directly with the human body in varied

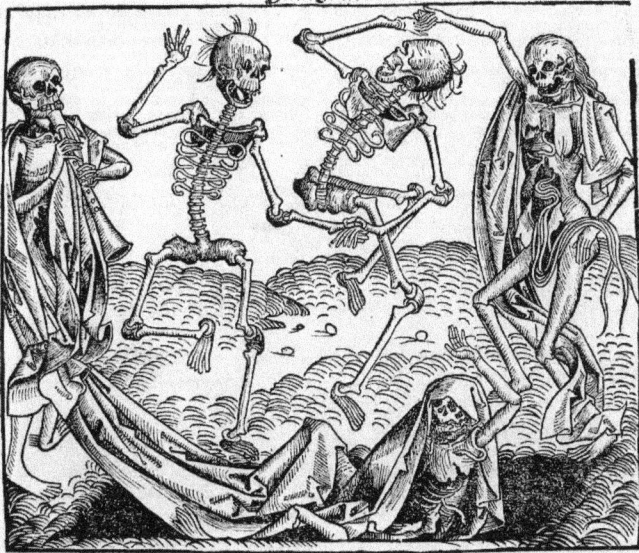

Figure 8: *Danse Macabre from the Nuremberg Chronicle (1493).*

states of sickness and health. Further, at this time, the importance of surgeons became more evident.

A theory put forth by Stephen O'Brien says the Black Death is likely responsible, through natural selection, for the high frequency of the CCR5-Δ32 genetic defect in people of European descent. The gene affects T cell function and provides protection against HIV, smallpox, and possibly plague, though for the last, no explanation as to how it would do that exists. This, however, is now challenged, given that the CCR5-Δ32 gene has been found to be just as common in Bronze Age tissue samples.

Architecture

The Black Death also inspired European architecture to move in two different directions: (1) a revival of Greco-Roman styles that, in stone and paint, expressed Petrarch's love of antiquity, and (2) a further elaboration of the Gothic style.[46] Late medieval churches had impressive structures centred on verticality, where one's eye is drawn up towards the high ceiling. The basic Gothic style was revamped with elaborate decoration in the late medieval period. Sculptors in Italian city-states emulated the work of their Roman forefathers while sculptors in northern Europe, no doubt inspired by the devastation they had witnessed, gave way to a heightened expression of emotion and an emphasis on individual differences.[47] A tough realism came forth in architecture as in literature. Images of intense sorrow, decaying corpses, and individuals with faults as well as virtues emerged. North of the Alps, painting reached a pinnacle of precise realism with Early Dutch painting by artists such as Jan van Eyck (c. 1390– by 1441). The natural world was reproduced in these works with meticulous detail whose realism was not unlike photography.[48]

Further reading

• Aberth, John, ed. *The Black Death: The Great Mortality of 1348–1350: A Brief History with Documents* (2005) excerpt and text search[49], with primary sources

• Benedictow, Ole J. *The Black Death 1346–1353: The Complete History* (2012) excerpt and text search[50]

• Borsch, Stuart J. *The Black Death in Egypt and England: A Comparative Study* (U of Texas Press, 2005) online[51]

• Britnell, R. H. "Feudal Reaction after the Black Death in the Palatinate of Durham," *Past & Present* No. 128 (Aug., 1990), pp. 28–47 in JSTOR[52], in England

• Byrne, Joseph P. *Encyclopedia of the Black Death* (2012) excerpt and text search[53]

• Cantor, Norman. *In the Wake of the Plague: The Black Death and the World it Made* (2001).

• Carmichael, Ann. *The Plague and the Poor in Renaissance Florence* (1986).

• Cohn, Samuel. "After the Black Death: Labour Legislation and Attitudes Towards Labour in Late-Medieval Western Europe," *Economic History Review* (2007) 60#3 pp. 457–485 in JSTOR[54]

• Deaux, George. *The Black Death, 1347* (1969)

• Gottfried, Robert S. *The Black Death: Natural and Human Disaster in Medieval Europe* (Simon & Schuster, 2010)

• Hatcher, John. *Plague, Population, and the English Economy, 1348–1530* (1977).

• Herlihy, David. *The Black Death and the Transformation of the West* (1997).

• Hilton, R. H. *The English Peasantry in the Late Middle Ages* (Oxford: Clarendon, 1974)

• Horrox, Rosemay, ed. *The black death* (Manchester University Press, 1994.)

• MacGregor, Kirk R. *A Comparative Study of Adjustments to Social Catastrophes in Christianity and Buddhism. The Black Death in Europe and the Kamakura Takeover in Japan As Causes of Religious Reform* (2011)

• Meiss, Millard. *Painting in Florence and Siena after the Black Death: the arts, religion, and society in the Mid-fourteenth century* (Princeton University Press, 1978)

• Platt, Colin. *King Death: The Black Death and Its Aftermath in Late Medieval England* (1996).

• Poos, Larry R. *A Rural Society after the Black Death: Essex, 1350–1525* (1991).

• Putnam, Bertha Haven. *The enforcement of the statutes of labourers during the first decade after the black death, 1349–1359*[55] (1908).

• Williman, Daniel, ed. *The Black Death: The Impact of the Fourteenth-Century Plague* (1982)

- Ziegler, Philip. *The black death* (1969), comprehensive older survey excerpt and text search[56]

Jewish Persecutions

Black Death Jewish persecutions

The **Black Death persecutions and massacres** were a series of violent attacks on Jewish communities blamed for an outbreak of the Black Death in Europe from 1348 to 1351.

History of persecutions

Christians despised Jews for their lack of conviction in Jesus Christ. The official church policy was to protect Jews because Jesus was born into the Jewish race. But in reality Jews were targets of Christian loathing. As the plague swept across Europe in the mid-14th century, annihilating nearly half the population, Jews were taken as scapegoats, likely because they were affected less than other people. Accusations spread that Jews had caused the disease by deliberately poisoning wells.[57,58]

The first massacres directly related to the plague took place in April 1348 in Toulon, France, where the Jewish quarter was sacked, and forty Jews were murdered in their homes, then in Barcelona.[59] In 1349, massacres and persecution spread across Europe, including the Erfurt massacre (1349), the Basel massacre, massacres in Aragon, and Flanders.[60,61] 2000 Jews were burnt alive on 14 February 1349 in the "Valentine's Day" Strasbourg massacre, where the plague had not yet affected the city. While the ashes smouldered, Christian residents of Strasbourg sifted through and collected the valuable possessions of Jews not burnt by the fires.[62] Many hundreds of Jewish communities were destroyed in this period. Within the 510 Jewish communities destroyed in this period, some members killed themselves to avoid the persecutions.[63] In the spring of 1349 the Jewish community in Frankfurth-am-Main was annihilated. This was followed by the destruction of Jewish communities in Mainz and Cologne. The 3000 strong Jewish population of Mainz initially defended

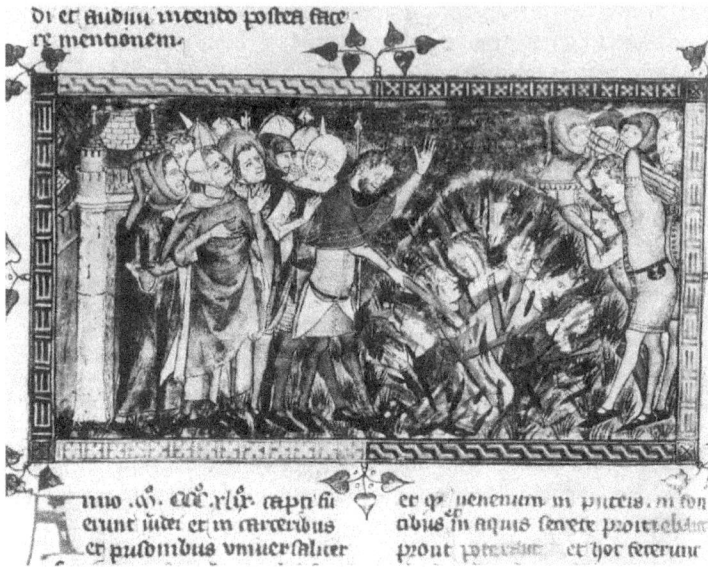

Figure 9: *Representation of a massacre of the Jews in 1349 Antiq-*
uitates Flandriae (Royal Library of Belgium manuscript 1376/77)

themselves and managed to hold off the Christian attackers. But the Christians
managed to overwhelm the Jewish ghetto in the end and killed all of its Jews.

At Speyer, Jewish corpses were disposed in wine casks and cast into the Rhine.
By the close of 1349 the worst of the pogroms had ended in Rhineland. But
around this time the massacres of Jews started rising near the Hansa town-
ships of the Baltic Coast and in Eastern Europe. By 1351 there had been 350
incidents of anti-Jewish pogroms and 60 major and 150 minor Jewish communities had been exterminated. All of this caused the eastward movement of
Northern Europe's Jewry to Poland and Russia, where they remained for the
next six centuries. King Casimir of Poland enthusiastically gave refuge and
protection to the Jews. The motives for this action is unclear. The king was
well disposed to Jews and had a Jewish mistress. He was also interested in
tapping the economic potential of the Jewry.

Reasons for relative Jewish immunity

There are many possible reasons why Jews were accused to be the cause for the
plague. One reason was because there was a general sense of anti-Semitism in
the 14th century. Jews were also isolated in the ghettos, which meant in some
places that Jews were less affected.[64] Additionally, there are many Jewish laws

that promote cleanliness: a Jew must wash his or her hands before eating bread and after using the bathroom, it was customary for Jews to bathe once a week before the Sabbath, a corpse must be washed before burial, and so on.

Government responses

In many cities the civil authorities either did little to protect the Jewish communities or actually abetted the rioters.[65] Pope Clement VI (the French born Benedictine, Pierre Roger) tried to protect the Jewish communities by two papal bulls (the first on July 6, 1348 and another 26 September 1348) saying that those who blamed the plague on the Jews had been "seduced by that liar, the Devil" and urging clergy to protect the Jews. In this, Clement was aided by the researches of his personal physician Guy de Chauliac who argued from his own treatment of the infected that the Jews were not to blame. Clement's efforts were in part undone by the newly elected Charles IV, Holy Roman Emperor making property of Jews killed in riots forfeit, giving local authorities a financial incentive to turn a blind eye.[66]

Aftermath

As the plague waned in 1350, so did the violence against Jewish communities. In 1351, the plague and the immediate persecution was over, though the background level of persecution and discrimination remained. Ziegler (1998) comments that "there was nothing unique about the massacres".[67] 20 years after the Black Death the Brussels massacre (1370) wiped out the Belgian Jewish community.[68]

Jewish tales of Black Death in Early Modern Period

Though told for nearly 350 years, there were no written accounts of the Black Death through Jewish tales until 1696, by Yiftah Yosef ben Naftali Hirts Segal Manzpach in the Mayse Nissim. Yuzpa Shammes, as he frequently was referred to, was a scribe and shammash of the Worms community for several decades. His accounts intend to show that the Jews were not idle but that they took action against inevitably becoming the scapegoat. Despite Yuzpa's assertion that the Jews fought against the massacres, there are contradicting accounts that claim that there was no evidence of "armed resistance".[69] These contradicting tales display the effect of oral tradition being manipulated to fit certain circumstances.

"Ordinary folk hated the Jews because they had served the merchants and aristocrats, and with their loans and with their capital, helped establish urban economy and the city's governing political and territorial independence. Further, the Jews had exploited artisans 'with loans at usurious rates'."[70] These reasons gave the "ordinary folk" the motive to kill the Jews because they were gaining political and social standings. Breuer also included that "others ... saw the massacres as the revenge of impoverished debtors against privileged elite of Jewish creditors."[71]

Second Plague

Second plague pandemic

The **second plague pandemic** is a major series of epidemics of the plague that started with the Black Death, which reached mainland Europe in 1348 and killed up to a half of the population of Eurasia in the next four years. Although it died out in most places, it became epizootic and recurred regularly until the nineteenth century. A series of major plagues occurred in the late 17th century and it recurred in some places until the 19th. After this a new strain of the bacterium appeared as the third pandemic.

Plague is caused by the bacterium *Yersinia pestis* which exists in the fleas of several species in the wild and particularly rats in human society. In an outbreak it may kill all its immediate hosts and thus die out, but remain active in other hosts which it does not kill and thereby cause a new outbreak years or decades later. It has several means of transmission and infection, including rats carried on board ships or vehicles, fleas hidden in grain, and in its more virulent forms is transmitted by blood and sputum directly between humans.

Overview

There have been three major outbreaks of plague. The Plague of Justinian in the 6th and 7th centuries is the first known attack on record, and marks the first firmly recorded pattern of bubonic plague. From historical descriptions, as much as 40% of the population of Constantinople died from the plague. Modern estimates suggest half of Europe's population died as a result of the plague before it disappeared in the 700s. After 750, major epidemic diseases did not appear again in Europe until the Black Death of the 14th century.[72]

The Second pandemic originated in or near China and was most likely spread by the Silk Road or by ship.[73] It may have reduced world population from an estimated 450 million down to 350–375 million by the year 1400.

World Distribution of Plague, 1998

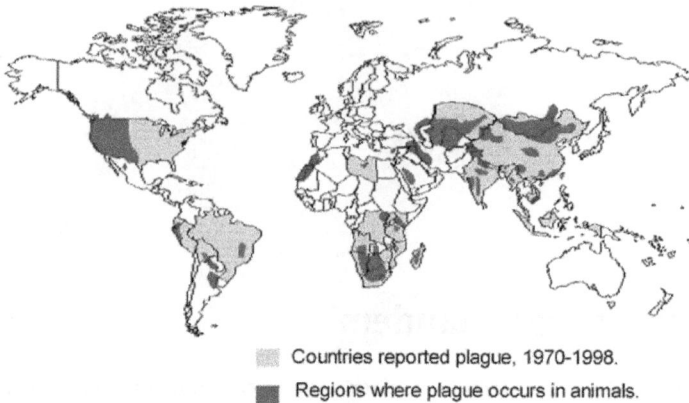

    Countries reported plague, 1970-1998.
    Regions where plague occurs in animals.

Figure 10: *Worldwide distribution of plague-infected animals 1998*

The plague returned at intervals with varying virulence and mortality until the early 19th century. In England, for example, the plague returned in
1360–63 killing 20% of Londoners and in 1369 killing 10–15%.[74] In the 17th-
century outbreaks were a series of "great plagues": the Great Plague of Seville
(1647–52); the Great Plague of London (1665–66); and the Great Plague of
Vienna (1679). In its virulent form, after the Great Plague of Marseille in
1720–22, the Great Plague of 1738 (which hit Eastern Europe), and the Russian plague of 1770–1772, it seems to have gradually disappeared from Europe
though lingering in Egypt and the Middle East. By the early 19th century, the
threat of plague had diminished, but it was quickly replaced by a new disease.
The Asiatic cholera was the first of several cholera pandemics to sweep through
Asia and Europe during the 19th and 20th centuries.[75]

The Third Pandemic hit China in the 1890s and devastated India, but was
largely contained in the east, though becoming endemic in the Western United
States. It still causes sporadic outbreaks.[73]

Black Death

Arab historians Ibn Al-Wardni and Almaqrizi believed the Black Death originated in Mongolia, and Chinese records show a huge outbreak in Mongolia in
the early 1330s. Europe was initially protected by a hiatus in the Silk Road,
but a 1347 Mongolian siege at Caffa—the last Italian outpost on the Crimean

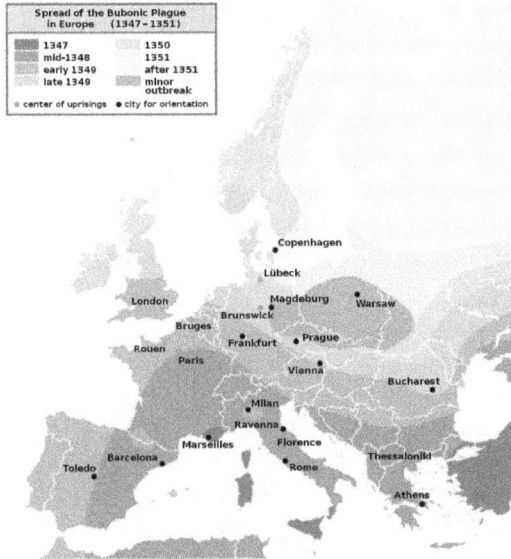

Figure 11: *Spread of the Black Death through Europe, 1347-51*

Peninsula—spread it to the defenders, who carried it back with them that winter. It arrived at Genoa and Venice in January 1348, while simultaneously spreading through Asia Minor and into Egypt. The bubonic form was described graphically in Florence in *The Decameron* and Guy de Chauliac also described the pneumonic form at Avignon. It rapidly spread to France and Spain, by 1349 was in England, in 1350 was afflicting eastern Europe and it reached the centre of Russia by 1351. In most parts it blew itself out within about three years, though only temporarily.

The 14th-century eruption of the Black Death had a drastic effect on Europe's population, irrevocably changing the social structure, and resulted in widespread persecution of minorities such as Jews, foreigners, beggars, and lepers (see Persecutions). The uncertainty of daily survival has been seen as creating a general mood of morbidity, influencing people to "live for the moment," as illustrated by Giovanni Boccaccio in *The Decameron* (1353).

There were large epidemics in China in 1331 and 1351-54 in Hopei, Shansi and other provinces which are considered to have killed between 50% and 90% of the local populations, running into tens of millions. However, there is no proof currently that these were caused by plague though there are indications for the second set of epidemics.[76]

Recurrence throughout Europe

The plague repeatedly returned to haunt Europe and the Mediterranean throughout the 14th to 17th centuries.[77] According to Biraben, plague was present somewhere in Europe in every year between 1346 and 1671.[78] Subsequent outbreaks, though severe, marked the retreat from most of Europe (18th century) and northern Africa (19th century).[79] According to Geoffrey Parker, "France alone lost almost a million people to plague in the epidemic of 1628–31."[80]

In 1466, perhaps 40,000 people died of plague in Paris.[74] During the 16th and 17th centuries, plague visited Paris for almost one year out of three.[81] The Black Death ravaged Europe for three years before it continued on into Russia, where the disease hit somewhere once every five or six years from 1350 to 1490.[82] Plague epidemics ravaged London in 1563, 1593, 1603, 1625, 1636, and 1665,[83] reducing its population by 10 to 30% during those years.[84] Over 10% of Amsterdam's population died in 1623–1625, and again in 1635–1636, 1655, and 1664.[85] There were 22 outbreaks of plague in Venice between 1361 and 1528. The plague of 1576–1577 killed 50,000 in Venice, almost a third of the population. Late outbreaks in central Europe included the Italian Plague of 1629–1631, which is associated with troop movements during the Thirty Years' War, and the Great Plague of Vienna in 1679. Over 60% of Norway's population died from 1348 to 1350. The last plague outbreak ravaged Oslo in 1654.

In the first half of the 17th century, a plague claimed some 1.7 million victims in Italy, or about 14% of the population.[86] In 1654, the Russian plague killed about 700,000 inhabitants[87,88]. In 1656, the plague killed about half of Naples' 300,000 inhabitants. More than 1.25 million deaths resulted from the extreme incidence of plague in 17th-century Spain.[89] The plague of 1649 probably reduced the population of Seville by half.[90] In 1709–1713, a plague epidemic that followed the Great Northern War (1700–1721, Sweden v. Russia and allies) killed about 100,000 in Sweden,[91] and 300,000 in Prussia.[90] The plague killed two-thirds of the inhabitants of Helsinki, and claimed a third of Stockholm's population. Western Europe's last major epidemic occurred in 1720 in Marseilles, in Central Europe the last major outbreaks happened during the plague during the Great Northern War, and in Eastern Europe during the Russian plague of 1770-1772 The plague ravaged much of the Islamic world. Plague was present in at least one location in the Islamic world virtually every year between 1500 and 1850.[92] Plague repeatedly struck the cities of North Africa. Algiers lost 30,000–50,000 to it in 1620–21, and again in 1654–57, 1665, 1691, and 1740–42.[93] Plague remained a major event in Ottoman society until the second quarter of the 19th century. Between 1701 and 1750, 37 larger and smaller epidemics were recorded in Constantinople, and

31 between 1751 and 1800. Baghdad has suffered severely from visitations of the plague, and sometimes two-thirds of its population has been wiped out.[94]

Some major outbreaks

Years	Place	Death estimates	Article/citation
1347–51	Europe	25,000,000	Black Death
1360–63	England	700–800,000	Black Death in England
1464–66	Paris	40,000	
1471	England	300–400,000	[95]
1479–80	England	400–500,000	[95]
1576–77	Venice	50,000	[96]
1596–99	Castile	500,000	[90]
1603–11	London	43,000	[97]
1620–21	Algiers	30–50,000	[93]
1628–31	France	1,000,000	[80]
1629–31	Italy	280,000	Italian plague of 1629–31
1647–52	South Spain	500,000	Great Plague of Seville
1654–55	Russia	700,000	[98,99]
1656–1657	Naples, Rome	150,000	Naples Plague
1664–1667	London	70–100,000	Great Plague of London
1679–80	Austria	76,000	Great Plague of Vienna
1681	Prague	83,000	
1689–1690	Baghdad	150,000	[94]
1704–10	Poland	75,000	Great Northern War plague outbreak
1709–13	Baltic	300–400,000	Great Northern War plague outbreak
1720s	Marseille	100,000	Great Plague of Marseille
1738–40	Hungary &c	50,000	Great Plague of 1738
1770s	Moscow	75,000	Russian plague of 1770–72
1772	Baghdad	70,000	[94]
1791	Egypt	300,000	[100]
1818–20	Tunisia		
1833–34	Baghdad	12,000	
1835–37	Alexandria	8,694	
1840s	Balkans		

1844	Egypt		100
1876	Baghdad	20,000	101

Disappearance

The second pandemic never became endemic in Europe. Most epidemics arrived with shipping from the near east and died out after a few years. But the pandemic died out progressively across Europe. One documented case was in 17th century London, where the first proper demographer, John Graunt, failed by just 5 years to see the last recorded death from plague, which happened in 1679, 14 years after the Great Plague of London. The reasons it died out totally are not well understood. It is tempting to think that the Great Fire of London the next year destroyed the hiding places of the rats in the roofs. Certainly there isn't a single plague death recorded "within the walls" after 1666. However the city by this time had spread well beyond the walls which contained most of the fire and most of plague cases happened beyond the limits of the fire. Probably more significant was the fact that all buildings after the fire were constructed of brick rather than wood and other flammable materials.

This pattern was broadly followed after major epidemics in northern Italy (1631), south and east Spain (1652), southern Italy and Genoa (1657), Paris (1668).

Appleby[102] considers six possible explanations:

1. People developed immunity.
2. Improvements in nutrition made people more resistant.
3. Improvements in housing, urban sanitation and personal cleanliness reduced the number of rats and rat fleas.
4. Change in dominant rat species. (The brown rat didn't arrive in London until 1727)
5. Quarantine methods improved in the 17th century.
6. Some rats developed immunity so fleas never left them in droves to humans, non-resistant rats were eliminated and this broke the cycle.

Probably most of these have some weight, but the answer is unclear.

The disappearance happened rather later in the Nordic and eastern European countries but there was a similar halt after major epidemics.

References

Bibliography

- Alexander, John T. (1980), *Bubonic Plague in Early Modern Russia: Public Health and Urban Disaster*[103], Oxford University Press, ISBN 978-0-19-515818-2
- Appleby, Andrew B. (1980), "The Disappearance of Plague: A Continuing Puzzle"[104], *The Economic History Review*, **33** (2): 161–173, doi: 10.1111/j.1468-0289.1980.tb01821.x[105], (Subscription required (help))
- Benedictow, Ole Jørgen (2004), *Black Death 1346-1353: The Complete History*[106], ISBN 978-1-84383-214-0
- Bray, R. S. (2004-04-29), *Armies of Pestilence: The Impact of Disease on History*[107], James Clarke & Co., ISBN 978-0-227-17240-7
- Shadwell, Arthur (1911), "Plague"[108], *Encyclopædia Britannica*, **21**, pp. 693–705
- Byrne, Joseph Patrick (2004), *The Black Death*, Westport, Connecticut: Greenwood Press
- Byrne, Joseph Patrick, ed. (2008), *Encyclopedia of Pestilence, Pandemics, and Plagues: A-M*[109], ABC-CLIO, ISBN 0-313-34102-8
- Davis, Robert C. (2003-12-05), *Christian Slaves, Muslim Masters: White Slavery in the Mediterranean, the Barbary Coast and Italy, 1500-1800*[110], Palgrave Macmillan, ISBN 978-0-333-71966-4
- Gottfried, Robert S. (1983), *The Black Death: Natural and Human Disaster in Medieval Europe*, London: Hale, ISBN 0-7090-1299-3
- Graunt, John (1759), *Collection of Yearly Bills of Mortality, from 1657 to 1758 Inclusive*[111]
- Harding, Vanessa (2002-06-20), *The Dead and the Living in Paris and London, 1500-1670*[112], Cambridge University Press, ISBN 978-0-521-81126-2
- Hays, J. N. (1998), *The Burdens of Disease: Epidemics and Human Response in Western History*[113], Rutgers University Press, ISBN 978-0-8135-2528-0
- Hays, J. N. (2005-12-31), *Epidemics And Pandemics: Their Impacts on Human History*[114], ABC-CLIO, ISBN 978-1-85109-658-9
- McNeill, William Hardy (1998), *Plagues and peoples*, Anchor, ISBN 978-0-385-12122-4
- Mikhail, Alan (2014), *The Animal in Ottoman Egypt*[115], OUP
- Issawi, Charles Philip (1988), *Fertile Crescent, 1800-1914: A Documentary Economic History*[116], Oxford University Press, ISBN 978-0-19-504951-0
- Parker, Geoffrey (2001-12-21), *Europe in Crisis: 1598-1648*[117], Wiley, ISBN 978-0-631-22028-2

- Porter, Stephen (2009-04-19), *The Great Plague*[118], Amberley Publishing, ISBN 978-1-84868-087-6
- Wade, Nicholas (31 October 2010), *Europe's Plagues Came From China, Study Finds*[119], The New York Times, retrieved 1 November 2010

External links

Media related to Plague, second pandemic at Wikimedia Commons

Third Plague

Third plague pandemic

Third Pandemic is the designation of a major bubonic plague pandemic that began in Yunnan province in China in 1855. This episode of bubonic plague spread to all inhabited continents, and ultimately more than 12 million people died in India and China, with 10 million people killed in India alone.[120] According to the World Health Organization, the pandemic was considered active until 1959, when worldwide casualties dropped to 200 per year.Wikipedia:Citation needed

The name refers to this pandemic being the third major bubonic plague outbreak known to western sources. The first was the Plague of Justinian, which ravaged the Byzantine Empire and surrounding areas in 541 and 542. The second was the Black Death, which killed at least one third of Europe's population in a series of expanding waves of infection from 1346 to 1353.

Casualty patterns indicate that waves of this late-19th-century/early-20th-century pandemic may have been from two different sources. The first was primarily bubonic and was carried around the world through ocean-going trade, through transporting infected persons, rats, and cargoes harboring fleas. The second, more virulent strain, was primarily pneumonic in character with a strong person-to-person contagion. This strain was largely confined to Asia, in particular Manchuria and Mongolia.

Pattern of the pandemic

The bubonic plague was endemic in populations of infected ground rodents in central Asia, and was a known cause of death among migrant and established human populations in that region for centuries. An influx of new people due to political conflicts and global trade led to the distribution of this disease throughout the world.

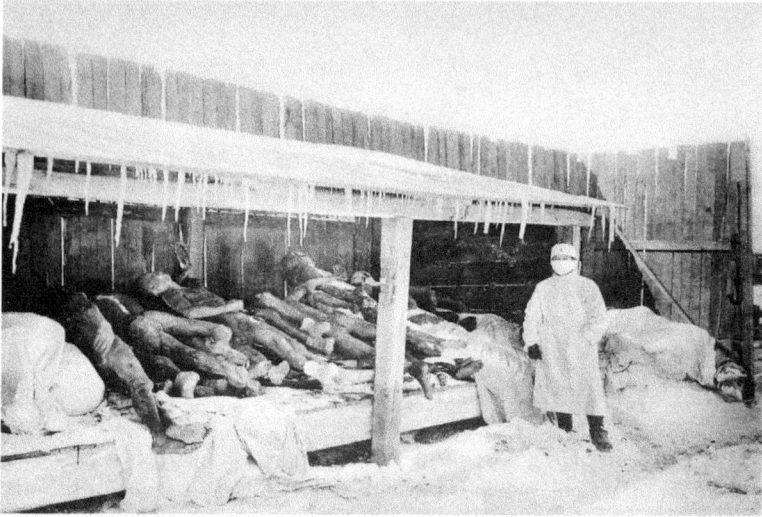

Figure 12: *Picture of Manchurian plague victims in 1910–1911*

Origin in Yunnan Province of China

A natural reservoir or nidus for plague is located in western Yunnan and is an ongoing health risk today. The third pandemic of plague originated in this area after a rapid influx of Han Chinese to exploit the demand for minerals, primarily copper, in the latter half of the eighteenth century. By 1850, the population had exploded to over 7 million people. Increasing transportation throughout the region brought people in contact with plague-infected fleas, the primary vector between the yellow-breasted rat (Rattus flavipectus) and humans. People brought the fleas and rats back into growing urban areas, where small outbreaks sometimes reached epidemic proportions. The plague spread further after disputes between Han Chinese and Hui Muslim miners in the early 1850s erupted into a violent uprising known as the Panthay rebellion, which led to further displacements (troop movements and refugee migrations). The outbreak of the plague helped recruit people into the Taiping Rebellion. In the latter half of the nineteenth century the plague began to appear in Guangxi and Guangdong provinces, Hainan Island, and later the Pearl River delta including Canton and Hong Kong. The plague was most likely brought from the interior of China to the coastal regions by traders in the growing and lucrative opium trade that began after about 1840.

In the city of Canton, beginning in March 1894, the disease killed 60,000 people in a few weeks. Daily water-traffic with the nearby city of Hong Kong rapidly spread the plague. Within two months, after 100,000 deaths, the death

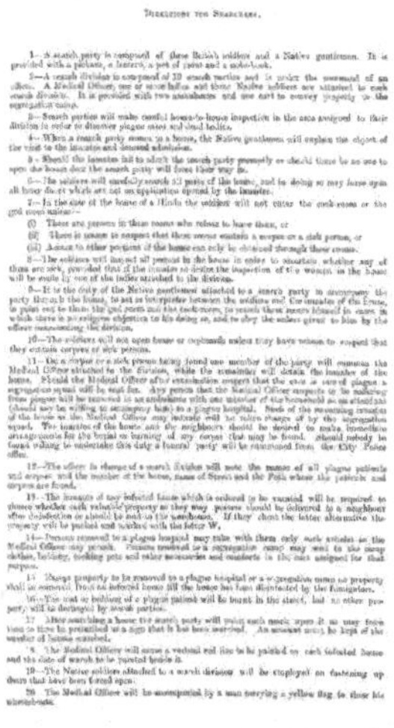

Figure 13: *Directions for searchers, Pune plague of 1897*

rates dropped below epidemic rates, although the disease continued to be endemic in Hong Kong until 1929.

Political impact in colonial India

Plague came to British India in 1896, most likely from Hong Kong where the epidemic had been festering since 1894. Over the next thirty years, the country would lose 12.5 million people to the disease. Almost all cases were bubonic, with only a very small percentage changing to pneumonic plague. (Orent, p. 185) The disease was initially seen in port cities, beginning with Bombay (now Mumbai), but later emerged in Pune, Kolkata, and Karachi (now in Pakistan). By 1899, the outbreak spread to smaller communities and rural areas in many regions of India. Overall, the impact of plague epidemics was greatest in western and northern India—in the provinces then designated as Bombay, Punjab, and the United Provinces—while eastern and southern India were not as badly affected.

The colonial government's measures to control the disease included quarantine, isolation camps, travel restrictions and the exclusion of India's traditional medical practices. Restrictions on the populations of the coastal cities were established by Special Plague Committees with overreaching powers, and enforced by the British military. Indians found these measures culturally intrusive and, in general, repressive and tyrannical. Government strategies of plague control underwent significant changes during 1898–1899. By that time, it was apparent that the use of force in enforcing plague regulations was proving counter-productive and, now that the plague had spread to rural areas, enforcement in larger geographic areas would be impossible. At this time, British health officials began to press for widespread vaccination using Waldemar Haffkine's plague vaccine, although the government stressed that inoculation was not compulsory. British authorities also authorized the inclusion of practitioners of indigenous systems of medicine into plague prevention programs.

Repressive government actions to control the plague led the Pune nationalists to criticise the government publicly. On 22 June 1897, the Chapekar brothers, young Pune Hindus, shot and killed Walter Charles Rand, an Indian Civil Services officer acting as Pune Special Plague Committee chairman, and his military escort, Lieutenant Ayerst. The action of the Chapekars was seen as terrorism. The government also found the nationalist press guilty of incitement. Independence activist Bal Gangadhar Tilak was charged with sedition for his writings as editor of the Kesari newspaper. He was sentenced to eighteen months rigorous imprisonment.

Public reaction to the health measures enacted by the British Indian state ultimately revealed the political constraints of medical intervention in the country. These experiences were formative in the development of India's modern public health services.Wikipedia:Citation needed

Global distribution

The network of global shipping ensured the widespread distribution of the disease over the next few decades. Recorded outbreaks include:

- Pakhoi, China 1882.
- Canton, China 1894.
- Hong Kong 1894.
- Taiwan, Japan 1896.
- Bombay Presidency, India 1896–1898.
- Calcutta, India 1898.
- Madagascar, 1898.
- Egypt, 1899.
- Manchuria, China 1899.
- Paraguay, 1899.
- South Africa, 1899–1902.
- Territory of Hawaii, 1899.[121]
- San Francisco, United States, 1900.
- Australia, 1900–1905.
- Russian Empire/Soviet Union, 1900–1927.

- Fukien Province, China 1901.
- Siam, 1904.
- Burma, 1905.
- Tunisia, 1907.
- Trinidad, Venezuela, Peru and Ecuador, 1908.
- Bolivia and Brazil, 1908.
- Cuba and Puerto Rico, 1912.

Each of these areas, as well as Great Britain, France, and other areas of Europe, continued to experience plague outbreaks and casualties until the 1950s. The last significant outbreak of plague associated with the pandemic occurred in Peru and Argentina in 1945.

Disease research

Researchers working in Asia during the "Third Pandemic" identified plague vectors and the plague bacillus. In 1894, in Hong Kong, Swiss-born French bacteriologist Alexandre Yersin isolated the responsible bacterium (*Yersinia pestis*) and determined the common mode of transmission. In 1898, French researcher Paul-Louis Simond demonstrated the role of fleas as a vector.

The disease is caused by a bacterium usually transmitted by the bite of fleas from an infected host, often a black rat. The bacteria are transferred from the blood of infected rats to the rat flea (*Xenopsylla cheopsis*). The bacillus multiplies in the stomach of the flea, blocking it. When the flea next bites a mammal, the consumed blood is regurgitated along with the bacillus into the bloodstream of the bitten animal. Any serious outbreak of plague in humans is preceded by an outbreak in the rodent population. During the outbreak, infected fleas that have lost their normal rodent hosts seek other sources of blood. The bacterium that causes this disease, *Yersinia pestis*, was named after Yersin. His discoveries led in time to modern treatment methods, including insecticides, the use of antibiotics and eventually plague vaccines.

The British colonial government in India pressed medical researcher Waldemar Haffkine to develop a plague vaccine. After three months of persistent work with a limited staff, a form for human trials was ready. On January 10, 1897 Haffkine tested it on himself. After the initial test was reported to the authorities, volunteers at the Byculla jail were used in a control test, all inoculated prisoners survived the epidemics, while seven inmates of the control group died. By the turn of the century, the number of inoculees in India alone reached four million. Haffkine was appointed the Director of the Plague Laboratory (now called Haffkine Institute) in Bombay.

Further reading

<templatestyles src="Template:Refbegin/styles.css" />

- ⬓ Media related to Plague, third pandemic at Wikimedia Commons
- Advisory Committee for Plague Investigations in India (1911), *Report On Plague Investigations In India, 1906-1910*[122]
- Gandhi, M. K. *The Plague Panic in South Africa*
- Gregg, Charles. *Plague: An Ancients Disease in the Twentieth Century.* Albuquerque, University of New Mexico Press, 1985.
- Kelly, John. *The Great Mortality: An Intimate History of the Black Death, the Most Devastating Plague of All Time.* New York: Harper-Collins Publishers, 2005. ISBN 0-06-000692-7.
- McNeill, William H. *Plagues and People.* New York: Anchor Books, 1976. ISBN 0-385-12122-9.
- Orent, Wendy. *Plague: The Mysterious Past and Terrifying Future of the World's Most Dangerous Disease.* New York: Free Press, 2004. ISBN 0-7432-3685-8.

External links

- Visual Representations of the Third Plague Pandemic[123]

Appendix

References

[1] http://www.medicalnewstoday.com/articles/206309.php

[2] Michael W. Dols, "The Second Plague Pandemic and Its Recurrences in the Middle East: 1347–1894" *Journal of the Economic Social History of the Orient* vol. 22 no. 2 (May 1979), 170–171.

[3] Wheelis, M. (2002). Biological Warfare at the 1346 Siege of Caffa. *Emerging Infectious Diseases, 8* (9), 971-975.

[4] Ping-ti Ho, "An Estimate of the Total Population of Sung-Chin China", in *Études Song*, Series 1, No 1, (1970) pp. 33–53.

[5]

[6] Suiyuan was a historical Chinese province that now forms part of Hebei and Inner Mongolia.

[7] McNeill, William H. (1976). *Plagues and People*. New York: Anchor Books.

[8] "At the beginning of October, in the year of the incarnation of the Son of God 1347, twelve Genoese galleys were fleeing from the vengeance which our Lord was taking on account of their nefarious deeds and entered the harbour of Messina. In their bones they bore so virulent a disease that anyone who only spoke to them was seized by a mortal illness and in no manner could evade death. ..Not only all those who had speech with them died, but also those who had touched or used any of their things. When the inhabitants of Messina discovered that this sudden death emanated from the Genoese ships they hurriedly ordered them out of the harbor and town. But the evil remained and caused a fearful outbreak of death." Michael Platiensis (1357), quoted in Johannes Nohl (1926). *The Black Death*, trans. C.H. Clarke. London: George Allen & Unwin Ltd., pp. 18–20.

[9] Secondary sources such as the *Cambridge History of Medieval England* often contain discussions of methodology in reaching these figures that are necessary reading for anyone wishing to understand this controversial episode in more detail.

[10] Rebecca Totaro, *Suffering in Paradise: The Bubonic Plague in English Literature from More to Milton* (Pittsburgh: Duquesne University Press: 2005), p. 26.

[11] Herlihy, *The Black Death and the Transformation of the West* (1997) Harvard University Press: Cambridge, MA, p. 29.

[12] July 22, 2014. The Black Death: Where We Are Now http://black-death-revisited.org

[13] Samuel K. Cohn, *The Black Death Transformed: Disease and Culture in Early Renaissance Europe* (London: Edward Arnold Publishers, 2002), 81.

[14] Scott, Susan and Duncan, Christopher. (2004). *Return of the Black Death: The World's Greatest Serial Killer* West Sussex; John Wiley and Sons.

[15] Bravata DM, Holty JE, Liu H, McDonald KM, Olshen RA, Owens DK (2006), Systematic review: a century of inhalational anthrax cases from 1900 to 2005, *Annals of Internal Medicine*; 144(4): 270–80.

[16] Hufthammer, Anne Karin and Walløe, Lars. 2012. Rats cannot have been intermediate hosts for *Yersinia pestis* during medieval plague epidemics in Northern Europe http://www.uib.no/filearchive/rats-plague-arch-akh-lw.pdf. Journal of Archaeological Science.

[17] Black Death plague now blamed on giant gerbils, not rats http://www.cbc.ca/news/technology/black-death-plague-now-blamed-on-giant-gerbils-not-rats-1.2969283

[18] Gerbils, Not Rats, May Have Caused Bubonic Plague, Study Finds http://abcnews.go.com/Health/gerbils-rats-caused-bubonic-plaque-study-finds/story?id=29192197

[19] Barbara A. Hanawalt, "Centuries of Transition: England in the Later Middle Ages," in Richard Schlatter, ed., *Recent Views on British History: Essays on Historical Writing since 1966* (Rutgers UP, 1984), pp 43–44, 58

[20] R.H. Hilton, *The English Peasantry in the Late Middle Ages* (Oxford: Clarendon, 1974)

[21] "The trend of recent research is pointing to a figure more like 45% to 50% of the European population dying during a four-year period. There is a fair amount of geographic variation. In Mediterranean Europe and Italy, the South of France and Spain, where plague ran

for about four years consecutively, it was probably closer to 75% to 80% of the population. In Germany and England, it was probably closer to 20%." Philip Daileader, *The Late Middle Ages*, audio/video course produced by The Teaching Company, 2007. Stéphane Barry and Norbert Gualde, in *L'Histoire* n° 310, June 2006, pp.45–46, say "between one-third and two-thirds"; Robert Gottfried (1983). "Black Death" in *Dictionary of the Middle Ages*, volume 2, pp.257–67, says "between 25 and 45 percent". Daileader, as above; Barry and Gualde, as above, Gottfried, as above. Norwegian historian Ole J. Benedictow ('The Black Death: The Greatest Catastrophe Ever', *History Today*, Volume 55 Issue 3 March 2005 (http://www.historytoday.com/ole-j-benedictow/black-death-greatest-catastrophe-ever); cf. Benedictow, *The Black Death 1346–1353: The Complete History*, Boydell Press (7 Dec. 2012), pp. 380ff.) suggests a death rate as high as 60%, or 50 million out of 80 million inhabitants.

[22] Jean Froissart, *Chronicles* (trans. Geoffrey Brereton, Penguin, 1968, corrections 1974), p. 111.

[23] Joseph Patrick Byrne (2004). *The Black Death.* , p. 64.

[24] According to Kelly (2005), "[w]oefully inadequate sanitation made medieval urban Europe so disease-ridden, no city of any size could maintain its population without a constant influx of immigrants from the countryside". The influx of new citizens facilitated the movement of the plague between communities and contributed to the longevity of the plague within larger communities. Kelly, John. *The Great Mortality, an Intimate History of the Black Death, the Most Devastating Plague of All Time.* NY: HarperCollins, 2005, p. 68

[25] Barry and Gualde 2006.

[26] Stéphane Barry and Norbert Gualde, "The Smallest Thing of History" (*La plus grande épidémie de l'histoire*, in *L'Histoire* n°310, June 2006, pp.45–46

[27] Bennett and Hollister, 329–330.

[28] http://voices.yahoo.com/the-devastating-impact-black-death-marriage-376886.html?cat=9

[29] Barbara A. Hanawalt, "centuries of Transition: England in the Later Middle Ages," in Richard Schlatter, ed., *Recent Views on British History: Essays on Historical Writing since 1966* (Rutgers UP, 1984), pp 43–44, 58

[30] http://spartacus-educational.com/YALDstatute.htm

[31] Gregory Clark, "The long march of history: Farm wages, population, and economic growth, England 1209–1869," *Economic History Review* 60.1 (2007): 97–135. online http://www.econstor.eu/bitstream/10419/31320/1/50512257X.pdf, page 36

[32] Samuel Cohn, "After the Black Death: Labour Legislation and Attitudes Towards Labour in Late-Medieval Western Europe," *Economic History Review* (2007) 60#3 pp. 457–485 in JSTOR https://www.jstor.org/stable/4502106

[33] David Nirenberg, *Communities of Violence*, 1998, .

[34] R.I. Moore *The Formation of a Persecuting Society*, Oxford, 1987

[35] Naomi E. Pasachoff, Robert J. Littman *A Concise History Of The Jewish People* 2005 – Page 154 "However, Jews regularly ritually washed and bathed, and their abodes were slightly cleaner than their Christian neighbors'. Consequently, when the rat and the flea brought the Black Death, Jews, with better hygiene, suffered less severely ..."

[36] Joseph P Byrne, *Encyclopedia of the Black Death* Volume 1 2012 – Page 15 "Anti–Semitism and Anti–Jewish Violence before the Black Death ... Their attention to personal hygiene and diet, their forms of worship, and cycles of holidays were off-puttingly different."

[37] Anna Foa *The Jews of Europe After the Black Death* 2000 Page 146 "There were several reasons for this, including, it has been suggested, the observance of laws of hygiene tied to ritual practices and a lower incidence of alcoholism and venereal disease"

[38] Richard S. Levy *Antisemitism* 2005 Page 763 "Panic emerged again during the scourge of the Black Death in 1348, when widespread terror prompted a revival of the well poisoning charge. In areas where Jews appeared to die of the plague in fewer numbers than Christians, possibly because of better hygiene and greater isolation, lower mortality rates provided evidence of Jewish guilt."

[39] Joseph P. Byrne, *The Black Death* (Westport, Conn.: Greenwood Press, 2004), 108.

[40] Steven A. Epstein, *An Economic and Social History of Later Medieval Europe, 1000–1500* (2009) p 182

[41] Katherine L. French, *The Good Women of the Parish: Gender and Religion After the Black Death* (U of Pennsylvania Press, 2011)

[42] Epstein, p 182

[43] J. M. Bennett and C. W. Hollister, *Medieval Europe: A Short History* (New York: McGraw-Hill, 2006), p. 372.

[44] Quotes from the Plague http://www.insecta-inspecta.com/fleas/bdeath/Quotes.html

[45] David Herlihy, *The Black Death and the Transformation of the West* (Cambridge, Mass.: Harvard University Press, 1997), 72.

[46] Bennett and Hollister, p. 374.

[47] Bennett and Hollister, p. 375.

[48] Bennett and Hollister, p. 376.

[49] https://www.amazon.com/Black-Death-Mortality-1348-1350-Documents/dp/031240087X/

[50] https://www.amazon.com/Black-Death-1346-1353-Complete-History/dp/1843832143/

[51] https://www.questia.com/library/118550983/the-black-death-in-egypt-and-england-a-comparative

[52] https://www.jstor.org/stable/651008

[53] https://www.amazon.com/Encyclopedia-Black-Death-Joseph-Byrne/dp/1598842536/

[54] https://www.jstor.org/stable/4502106

[55] https://books.google.com/books?hl=en&lr=&id=ek8pAAAAYAAJ

[56] https://www.amazon.com/Black-Death-Philip-Ziegler/dp/006171898X/

[57] Anna Foa *The Jews of Europe After the Black Death* 2000 Page 146 "There were several reasons for this, including, it has been suggested, the observance of laws of hygiene tied to ritual practices and a lower incidence of alcoholism and venereal disease"

[58] Richard S. Levy *Antisemitism* 2005 Page 763 "Panic emerged again during the scourge of the Black Death in 1348, when widespread terror prompted a revival of the well poisoning charge. In areas where Jews appeared to die of the plague in fewer numbers than Christians, possibly because of better hygiene and greater isolation, lower mortality rates provided evidence of Jewish guilt."

[59] Anna Foa *The Jews of Europe after the black death* 2000 p. 13 "This was the context in which the Plague made its appearance in 1348. THE BLACK DEATH The Plague was not unknown in ... The first massacres took place in April 1348 in Toulon, where the Jewish quarter was raided and forty Jews were murdered in their homes. Shortly afterward, violence broke out in Barcelona and in other Catalan cities."

[60] *Codex Judaica: chronological index of Jewish history*; p. 203 Máttis Kantor - 2005 "1349 The Black Death massacres swept across Europe. .. The Jews were savagely attacked and massacred, by sometimes hysterical mobs — normal social order had ..."

[61] John Marshall *John Locke, Toleration and Early Enlightenment Culture*; p. 376 2006 "The period of the Black Death saw the massacre of Jews across Germany, and in Aragon, and Flanders",

[62] See Stéphane Barry and Norbert Gualde, «La plus grande épidémie de l'histoire» ("The greatest epidemic in history"), in *L'Histoire* magazine, n° 310, June 2006, p. 47

[63] Durant, Will. "The Renaissance" Simon and Schuster (1953), page 730–731,

[64] Joseph P Byrne, *Encyclopedia of the Black Death* Volume 1 2012—Page 15 "Anti–Semitism and Anti–Jewish Violence before the Black Death .. Their attention to personal hygiene and diet, their forms of worship, and cycles of holidays were off-puttingly different."

[65] Howard N. Lupovitch *Jews and Judaism in world history* p92—2009 "In May 1349, the city fathers of Brandenburg passed a law a priori condemning Jews of well poisoning: Should it become evident and proved by reliable men that the Jews have caused or will cause in the future the death of Christians,..."

[66] Howard N. Lupovitch *Jews and Judaism in world history* p. 92 2009 "On July 6, 1349, Pope Clement tried to curb anti-Jewish violence by issuing a papal bull. Its effectiveness was limited by the Holy Roman Emperor Charles IV, who made arrangements for the disposal of Jewish property in the event of a ..."

[67] Philip Ziegler *The Black Death* 1998 "The persecution of the Jews waned with the Black Death itself; by 1351 all was over. Save for the horrific circumstances of the plague which provided the incentive and the background, there was nothing unique about the massacres."

[68] *The Shengold Jewish Encyclopedia* Mordecai Schreiber—2011 "In 1370, after the Black Death, the brutal Brussels Massacre wiped out the Belgian Jewish community"

[69] *Die Chronik des Mathias von Neuenburg*, 1955. "While a Christian chronicler reports that during the pogrom of March 1, 1349, the beleaguered Jews of Worms set fire to their own houses, as may have happened elsewhere, there is no evidence of armed resistance."

[70] *The 'Black Death' and Antisemitism*, 1998. "Ordinary folk hated the Jews because they had served the merchants and aristocrats, and with their loans and with their capital, helped establish urban economy and the city's governing political and territorial independence. Further, the Jews had exploited artisans 'with loans at usurious rates'."

[71] Samuel K. Cohen Jr. *The Black Death and the Burning of Jews*, 2007. "others ... saw the massacres as the revenge of impoverished debtors against privileged elite of Jewish creditors."

[72] Hays 2005, p. 23.

[73] Wade 2010.

[74] Britannica 1911.

[75] " Cholera's seven pandemics http://www.cbc.ca/health/story/2008/05/09/f-cholera-outbreaks. html". CBC News. 2 December 2008.

[76] McNeill 1998.

[77] Parker 2009, p. 25.

[78] Hays 1998, p. 58.

[79] Hays 2005, p. 46.

[80] Parker 2001, p. 7.

[81] Harding 2002, p. 25.

[82] Byrne 2004, p. 62.

[83] Harding 2002, p. 24.

[84] " Plague in London: spatial and temporal aspects of mortality http://www.history.ac.uk/cmh/ epitwig.html", J. A. I. Champion, *Epidemic Disease in London, Centre for Metropolitan History Working Papers Series*, No. 1 (1993).

[85] Geography, climate, population, economy, society http://history.wisc.edu/sommerville/351/ 351-012.htm . J.P.Sommerville.

[86] Karl Julius Beloch, *Bevölkerungsgeschichte Italiens*, volume 3, pp. 359–360.

[87] Collins S. (1671) *The Present State of Russia http://ir.uiowa.edu/cgi/viewcontent.cgi? article=1000&context=history_pubs*. Edited by Marshall T. Poe, 2008

[88] Медовиков П. Е. (1854) *Историческое значение царствования Алексея Михайловича http://elib.shpl.ru/nodes/20688#page/82/mode/inspect/zoom/6*

[89] The Seventeenth-Century Decline http://libro.uca.edu/payne1/payne15.htm, S. G. Payne, *A History of Spain and Portugal*

[90] Bray 2004, p. 72.

[91] Alexander 1980, p. 21.

[92] Byrne 2008, p. 519.

[93] Davis 2003, p. 18.

[94] Issawi 1988, p. 99.

[95] Gottfried 1983, p. 131.

[96] Bray 2004, p. 71.

[97] Graunt 1759.

[98] Collins S. (1671) *The Present State of Russia http://ir.uiowa.edu/cgi/viewcontent.cgi?article= 1000&context=history_pubs*. Edited by Marshall T. Poe, 2008

[99] Медовиков П. Е. (1854) *Историческое значение царствования Алексея Михайловича http://elib.shpl.ru/nodes/20688#page/82/mode/inspect/zoom/6*

[100] Mikhail 2014, p. 43.

[101] Hirsh 1883, p. 513.

[102] Appleby 1980.

[103] https://books.google.com/books?id=IcljzNyv4EgC&pg=PA21

[104] https://www.jstor.org/discover/10.2307/2595837

[105] //doi.org/10.1111/j.1468-0289.1980.tb01821.x

[106] https://www.amazon.com/Black-Death-1346-1353-Complete-History/dp/1843832143

[107] https://books.google.com/books?id=djPWGnvBm08C&pg=PA72

[108] https://en.wikisource.org/wiki/1911_Encyclop%C3%A6dia_Britannica/Plague
[109] https://books.google.com/books?id=5Pvi-ksuKFIC&pg=PA519&dq#v=onepage&q=&f=false
[110] https://books.google.com/books?id=5q9zcB3JS40C&pg=PA18
[111] https://archive.org/details/collectionyearl00hebegoog
[112] https://books.google.com/books?id=JCPXfSUlUV8C&pg=PA25
[113] https://books.google.com/books?id=iMHmn9c38QgC&pg=PA58
[114] https://books.google.com/books?id=GyE8Qt-kS1kC&pg=PA46
[115] https://books.google.com/books?id=hfMEAQAAQBAJ
[116] https://books.google.com/books?id=F2TGkO7G43oC&pg=PA99
[117] https://books.google.com/books?id=qy8y8rHgucoC&pg=PA7
[118] https://books.google.com/books?id=x2EBkPNnUXEC&pg=PA25
[119] https://www.nytimes.com/2010/11/01/health/01plague.html
[120] Infectious Diseases: Plague Through History http://www.sciencemag.org/cgi/content/full/321/5890/773, sciencemag.org
[121] https://scholarsbank.uoregon.edu/xmlui/bitstream/handle/1794/7694/Bailey_Kevin_thesis2007.pdf?sequence=1
[122] https://books.google.com/books?id=5ME8AAAAIAAJ&pg=RA1-PA13
[123] http://www.crassh.cam.ac.uk/programmes/visual-representations-of-the-third-plague-pandemic

Article Sources and Contributors

The sources listed for each article provide more detailed licensing information including the copyright status, the copyright owner, and the license conditions.

Black Death migration *Source:* https://en.wikipedia.org/w/index.php?oldid=842903912 *License:* Creative Commons Attribution-Share Alike 3.0 *Contributors:* 99percentNog1percentNig, AlbertBickford, Allens, Anbu121, AnneTG, Antandrus, Arthena, AxelBoldt, BD2412, Bilsonius, C xong, Catalaalatac, Cement37843, Chris55, ChrisGualtieri, ClueBot NG, Doug Weller, EconomicHisorianinTraining, Excirial, Gary, Gilliam, Good Olfactory, Granola flakes, HaeB, Headbomb, Hibernian, Hmains, I dream of horses, Jagged 85, Jhoffa232, Ketiltrout, Khazar2, Llywrch, Me, Myself, and I are Here, Metahacker, Morlick, MusikAnimal, Naviguessor, NawlinWiki, Rich Farmbrough, Rjwilmsi, Rrburke, Ruslik0, Satani, Skamecrazy123, Stars4change, Tom.Reding, Trappist the monk, Twas Now, Uskill, Vanamonde93, Widr, Ylai, Your mums dads mum, 55 anonymous edits 1

Theories of the Black Death *Source:* https://en.wikipedia.org/w/index.php?oldid=847765104 *License:* Creative Commons Attribution-Share Alike 3.0 *Contributors:* A million reasons, Adam Bishop, AdventurousSquirrel, Ananiujitha, Arakunem, Archaeogenetics, Art LaPella, Auric, BBuchbinder, BRPever, CASSIOPEIA, Carolina cotton, Catalaalatac, CelestialStar14, Champion97, Chris55, ClueBot NG, CowboySpartan, Crusader8968, Difu Wu, DocWatson42, Donner60, Doug Weller, Dunks58, Excirial, Fayenatic london, Flyer22 Reborn, Fnielsen, Gary, Jachyra-NoSan, Jakelorich, Jdrum00, Jeremiah Y, Jonesey95, Jusdafax, K6ka, Kilmer-san, Kogmaw, Lucobrat, Oshwah, PierceG, Quenhitran, Rjwilmsi, Rushbugled13, Ruslik0, Satani, Skamecrazy123, Sailboatd2, Septrillion, Sietse Snel, Sketchmoose, Spencerk, Stone, The Thing That Should Not Be, Versus22, Wetman, Wiae, Widr, Wyrtian, Yikeshehehe, Ylai, ÀrdRuadh21, 92 anonymous edits 7

Consequences of the Black Death *Source:* https://en.wikipedia.org/w/index.php?oldid=847137411 *License:* Creative Commons Attribution-Share Alike 3.0 *Contributors:* Aegis100, Ajayay, Asdfghjklqwertyuiop1234, Asipppiakds, Blue Edits, BrxBrx, C.J. Griffin, CAPTAIN RAJU, CASSIOPEIA, CLCStudent, CambridgeBayWeather, Cellorelio, Checkingfax, Chris the speller, Classicwiki, ClueBot NG, Cortagravatas, Crystallizedcarbon, CyanoTex, Daisyy.thomass, DatGuy, David.moreno72, DavidLeighEllis, Dawnseeker2000, Dbachmann, Dcirovic, DemocraticLuntz, Diptanshu Das, Donner60, Ehrenkater, Esszet, Excirial, FeralOink, Fmadd, FoCuSandLcArN, Fobbs, GSS, Gilliam, Gulumeemee, GünniX, Happysailor, Headbomb, Hello71, Here2help, Hillbillyholiday, Hmainsbot1, Home Lander, Jim1138, Joeyinthehouse, Joshua Scott, K6ka, KGirlTrucker81, KNHaw, L3X1, Magesticowlsareawesome, Materialscientist, Nihlus, Niyaa More, ODST-K74, OcarinaOfTime, Optakeover, Orphan Wiki, Oshwah, PJsg1011, PainMan, Passengerpigeon, Philip Trueman, PlyrStar93, PriceDL, Quinton Feldberg, Qzd, RA0808, RileyBugz, Ruby2502, Ruslik0, Sabrebd, Samf4u, Serols, Shellwood, Siddiqsazzad001, Simplexity22, Stefanomione, SuperTurboChampionshipEdition, TheGracefulSlick, Thelost byte, ToBeFree, Tom.Reding, Tomaso rall, Vanstrat, Wavehunter, Wikipelli, Wikishovel, Will-B, Wisedog1010, Yes my sir, Zerolevel, Zppix, Île flottante, 263 anonymous edits 17

Black Death Jewish persecutions *Source:* https://en.wikipedia.org/w/index.php?oldid=853142723 *License:* Creative Commons Attribution-Share Alike 3.0 *Contributors:* AddWittyNameHere, Allens, Bender235, Byteflush, Caeden.M, ClueBot NG, DavidPreston, Discospinster, Dontreader, Editor75937965959, Felix Folio Secundus, FreeRangeFrog, Gilliam, GreenC, Gruzinim, Harizotoh9, In ictu oculi, Jami430, Jcurci12, Jeff G., JosephusOfJerusalem, Jprg1966, KH-1, Kaalesia, Kakasprincess, Kuivsto1utogomen, Lipsquid, MShabazz, Magioladitis, Marcocapelle, Mariolis MG, Materialscientist, Nimetapoeg, Oshwah, PhilipC, Ruslik0, Sabrebd, ShawntheGod, SkyWarrior, Smalljim, Sofia Bibars, Steveodinkirk, Vargob, בן 68 anonymous edits 31

Second plague pandemic *Source:* https://en.wikipedia.org/w/index.php?oldid=841811586 *License:* Creative Commons Attribution-Share Alike 3.0 *Contributors:* Alitkumar, AndrewOne, Beland, Bgwhite, Chris55, Cleph, ClueBot NG, Da Vynci, Dcirovic, Djr13, Dlpflipper, DocWatson42, Drbignosejude, LlywelynII, Look2See1, MShabazz, Marcos110202, Me, Myself, and I are Here, Richard Arthur Norton (1958-), Roxy the dog, Serols, VexorAbVikipædia, Wikisanchez, Мечников, 14 anonymous edits 35

Third plague pandemic *Source:* https://en.wikipedia.org/w/index.php?oldid=852723601 *License:* Creative Commons Attribution-Share Alike 3.0 *Contributors:* 0704monochrome, Ajpolino, Arch dude, Bangee ca〜enwiki, Bellerophon, Bender235, Benjwong, Binksternet, CDN99, CanisRufus, Cgingold, Chris55, Chrissymad, ClueBot NG, Craig Pemberton, Cratai42, D6, DBaba, Da Vynci, Dcirovic, Djr13, Dlpflipper, DocWatson42, Drbignosejude, Dr-philharmonic, FirstPrinciples, Gabriel Kielland, Gerry Lynch, Good Olfactory, GraemeLeggett, Grahamec, HarryHenryGebel, Hugo999, IQ125, Iffy6, Immunize, Investigation11111, JMagalhães, Jarble, Jonathan Drain, Jtamad, JuniperisCommunis, Karl Andrews, Kbailey1, Khazar2, KrmartinCA, Lchiarav, Look2See1, Luca Edd Fike, MPS1992, Magafuzula, Magioladitis, Maury Markowitz, Max72Loew, Miles530, Monkey Bounce, Mr Stephen, Place Clichy, Prisencolin, Richard Arthur Norton (1958-), Riffle, Rjwilmsi, RodC, Ruslik0, Rédacteur Tibet, S3000, Salvadorjo〜enwiki, Sam Hocevar, Sinistrum, Sjö, Smyth, Stbalbach, Steffen, Stillwaterising, The Average Wikipedian, Tim!, Tom.Reding, Tpbradbury, Vmenkov, WBardwin, WarriorsPride6565, Wavelength, Wetman, Wikisanchez, William Avery, Winterst, Woohookitty, Yogesh Khandke, 自拍子花子, 67 anonymous edits 43

Image Sources, Licenses and Contributors

The sources listed for each image provide more detailed licensing information including the copyright status, the copyright owner, and the license conditions.

License

Index